MULTIPLE SCLEROSIS,
THE HORRENDOUS, NOTORIOUS, UNINVITED, INTRUDER

BY

E. C. McCOLLUM-FLANIGAN

This book is a work of non-fiction. Names and places have been changed to protect the privacy of all individuals. The events and situations are true.

© 2004 by E. C. McCollum-Flanigan. All rights reserved.

No part of this book may be reproduced, stored in a retrieval system, or transmitted by any means, electronic, mechanical, photocopying, recording, or otherwise, without written permission from the author.

ISBN: 1-4140-1570-4 (e-book)
ISBN: 1-4140-1571-2 (Paperback)

Library of Congress Control Number: 2003097605

This book is printed on acid free paper.

Printed in the United States of America
Bloomington, IN

1stBooks - rev. 01/24/04

ACKNOWLEDGEMENTS.........DEDICATION

PSALM 145: 14
The LORD upholds all those who fall, and lifts up all those who are bowed down.

This book is dedicated to all dear persons and their care-givers/care-takers, who suffer with Multiple Sclerosis.

Today there are many, many individuals and companies, that raise and designate funds to finance the research of discovering a cure for this debilitating disease of Multiple Sclerosis. A discovered cure will be a miracle from GOD, through HIS guidance with medical research. However, many who suffer with Multiple Sclerosis, including myself, will be a lot more content, if there were medications to ease and relieve the day to day malfunctions of the critical malady. We will gladly take a daily dosage of any approved medication, and know that we will have a non-suffering wonderful day.

My desire is to share some vital aspects of most of my personal experiences, that have caused me to change areas in my lifestyle. I delight in sharing my personal experiences to help others who have been diagnosed with Multiple Sclerosis, and those who are undergoing Central and Peripheral Nervous Systems screenings, and seeking diagnoses for malfunctions. My main goal is to let others know that they are not alone in any form or fashion, with this MS massive interferences.

In gratitude, I receive so much useful information from the "National Multiple Sclerosis Society," and others. Therefore, I make acknowledgements to its physicians, nurses, technicians and all medical personnel, counselors, phone call assistants and advocates, contributing writers, shared testimonies, and all contributors that I am mistakenly omitting, from the "National and Local Multiple Sclerosis Journals.

I fully give credits to others, if and when facts in this book appear to sound like something copied, and I have reused someone else's information. Of course, the Definition Section, was essentially paraphrased in order to share the specific meaning, as closely as `possible of the Multiple Sclerosis definition. Trust me, I have not used plagiarism. I am a confirmed reference seeker. Therefore, I have/am researching Multiple Sclerosis constantly. Thereby, I feel that I am able to translate most of the factual information that I have acquired. This is not to say that Multiple Sclerosis is easy to explain or describe. It is very difficult to explain and describe. But, just think about this. What is easy about the Multiple Sclerosis intruder? Easiness and simplicity are not in its game plan or strategies of attack.

This book is from my heart, and my thoughts, regardless of how it appears. Yes, I tend to get redundant too often. One old cliché states that in many areas of life, "You really have to be there to experience the ups and downs of what really goes on." I fully agree with that about Multiple Sclerosis. No two cases are the same, nor can the true experiences be described to the fullest one hundred percent without a lessened description.

No, I am not exaggerating on any particular sentences that I have written in this book.

They are not exaggerations. My mission is to try to tell it like it was/is for me. I was frank and honest in writing this book. Once, I would have been really embarrassed in sharing some of the predicaments and situations that I had experienced. I probably would have used omissions, and used options to camouflage parts of the real situations. Today, I am not ashamed of what I had to say in order to be exact as possible, and try to relate and help others know that those embarrassing MS consequences do happen.

I make further acknowledgements and dedications to my family and friends. I am not sharing photos, by my choice. Anyway, sorting and choosing photos would have taken me forever to choose the ones that I would have decided to publish. (I am loaded down with family photos and videos.)

I realize that photos and identifying recognition of each photo is definitely what helps to sell books. Yes, I do want to sell my publication. No, I am not selfish. I do not want to embarrass my family and friends, and they do know that I have some sharings about them too, in order to help bring full circle to my experiences. Do you know what? Some readers, that I speculate on, will simply identify who I am by the common things and circumstances that I have shared. That will be just fine with me, because our lives have gratefully crossed paths too.

Thank you for understanding my inner thoughts on the Multiple Sclerosis, and the specific Multiple Sclerosis enemy that I refer about. I join other writers who publish non-photo editions.

Please see us in Books Two! Just think, it is always interesting to get a mental image without visuals of whomever one is reading about.

I apologize for any unknown offenses that I have referred too, to anyone.

MY ACKNOWLEDGEMENTS and DEDICATION to ALL!

I. OPENING POEM

MULTIPLE SCLEROSIS CURE

Many MS patients are unable
Unfortunately to do,
Life's daily functions and occupations
That once were complete and through.
Independent studies, research, and
Perseverance is concrete,
Lending compassions for sufferers
Endlessly waiting for relief.

Systems will not fail, a
Cure is on the way,
LORD, hear our prayers and answer
Eternally today.
Rising costs are factors
On which research depends,
SAVIOR, do not pass us by
Into a long waiting trend.
Scientists are truly experimenting,

Continuously striving for sure.
Using various control substances
Researching for a cure, very
Effectively.

E. G. Mc-FLANIGAN

TABLE OF CONTENTS

PSALM 86:6
Give ear, O LORD, unto my prayer; and attend to the voice of my supplications.

ACKNOWLEDGEMENTS.........DEDICATION		iii
I.	OPENING POEM	vii
II.	INTRODUCTION.........DEFINITION	xi
III.	MINI-AUTOBIOGRAPHY	1
IV.	SOMETHING IS DEFINITELY WRONG	7
V.	ENDURANCE FOR A DIAGNOSIS	9
VI.	DIAGNOSIS AND CONSEQUENCES	13
VII.	MEDICAL DISABILITY RETIREMENT	17
VIII.	EMERGENCY HOSPITALIZATION	25
IX.	PHYSICAL STRENGTHS AND WEAKNESSES	43
	A. ACHES...PAINS...NERVE DAMAGES...MUSCLE TIGHTNESSES	46
	B. DENTAL	47
	C. VISION	49
	D. INSOMNIA	50

	E. INCONTINENCE/BLADDER DYSFUNCTION...............	53
	F. IRRITABLE BOWEL SYNDROME......................	58
	G. ALTERNATIVE…HOLISTIC…PROGRAMS................	63
X.	EMOTIONAL ROLLER COASTER.........................	69
XI.	FINANCIAL ADJUSTMENTS	83
XII.	SEXUALITY	89
XIII.	SPIRITUALITY AND MUCH GRATITUDE..................	91
XIV.	FAMILY—LOVING GRAND CHILDREN—CHURCH FRIENDS SOCIAL FRIENDS MULTIPLE SCLEROSIS SUPPORT GROUP	93
	LOVING GRAND CHILDREN............................	97
	CHURCH FAMILY FRIENDS............................	100
	MULTIPLE SCLEROSIS SUPPORT GROUP	101
XV.	PESSIMISTIC VERSUS OPTIMISTIC REALITIES...........	105
XVI.	THE PRESENT AND LIFE STYLE CHANGES	109
XVII.	CLOSING POEM.....................................	115
	CREDITS	117
	ABOUT THE AUTHOR	121

PSALM 37:34
DON'T BE IMPATIENT FOR THE LORD TO ACT!

II. INTRODUCTION.........DEFINITION

<u>PSALM 59:1</u> Deliver me from mine enemies, O GOD…
<u>PSALM 62:1</u> Truly my soul waited upon GOD: from HIM cometh my salvation.

    My loving and late father sometimes had a comical saying to guests.
    "Stay a week, or stay to you get weak!" Multiple Sclerosis does both. It stays until the weeks turn into years, and of course, by that time, one has become weak, weaker, and very often, weakest.
    Multiple Sclerosis, known commonly as MS, is a chronic inflammatory disease of the Central Nervous System (CNS), the brain and the spinal cord. Naturally, the Peripheral Nervous System (PNS) is also affected. The inflammations usually cause swelling around the blood vessels in the brain and spinal cord. The disease damages the myelin sheath, the insulating material that surrounds and protects the nerve fibers in the brain, spinal cord, and the optic nerves. When any extremely minute part of the myelin sheath is distorted, or disturbed, nerve impulses are interrupted. Those interruptions make the nerve signals move very slowly or not at all. Those interruptions range from slight to chronic malfunctions. The myelin usually is so severely scarred, that the nerves fail to recognize the mobility stimuli. The myelin is lost in multiple areas, leaving plaques (scars) called

sclerosis. That is how the name, "Multiple Sclerosis", came to be known. Sclerosis prevents the brain and spinal cord from coordinating and working normally.

Medically, and presently, the exact causes and cure are unknown. It is thought to be an autoimmune disease. It is definitely not contagious. It is not directly inherited, but there may be some genetic factors. Eventually, and probably through DNA screenings, pertinent factors will be identified.

MS is characterized as; "relapsing-remitting," "primary progressive", "secondary progressive", "progressive relapsing", and "remissions or recovery". Damages in any one will cause some forms of exacerbations presently, there is not a cure, but there are some injections that can slow down the rate of relapses. The exacerbations may be associated with plaques that prevent conduction of nerve impulses in the CNS. That is how the common lingo of MS is coined to me, "the uninvited intruder". It comes in frequently, disguised, and unscheduled, for a while. It finds a good hiding place, causes chaos, and discord to the maximum. It breaks into one's body and very uninvited, without remorse, takes over to destroy everything possible, like it owns the place.

With MS, it is what sometimes cannot be seen for periods of time that hurts.

The sneaky, incredible, MS intruder is very busy and active, even when one feels well. It is the master of disguise, until it is ready to reveal its visual damages to the patients and others.

Recorded history of MS began in 1868, when a French neurologist, Dr. Jean- Martin Charcot (1825-1893), (MS Journal) wrote a complete medical description of the disease and the effected changes in the brain that accompany it.

No two cases of MS are alike. The disease affects each person on a very individual level. However, there are lots of common characteristics among patients. The validity of the various difficulties of individual diagnosis of MS proves the broad range of characteristics of the disease. Unfortunately, but realistically, most people will experience some levels of obvious disabilities in the years following the onset of MS.

MS can be a very progressive deteriorating disease. It generally gets worse with time. The needs of people increase over time. It is recommended that patients regularly be re-assessed. The "National MS Society", is the largest organization fighting for the rights for professional people, present patients, as well as those suffering with MS who have been overlooked.

MS attacks all people. However, most individuals are diagnosed between the ages of 20 through 40 years old. There are more females diagnosed than there are males diagnosed.

The disease is more common among Caucasians than other races. This may be an invalid statistic, due to the fact that thousands of person's world wide, may have not been accurately tested, or probably have not been tested at all for their Central Nervous System ailments. This default has most likely been caused by lack of finance and lack of medical technology in areas for individuals. It is such a complicated camouflaging disease to diagnose because its presentation may imitate other diseases. The National Multiple Sclerosis Society estimates that there are approximately 3 million people with MS worldwide, and about 350,000 in the United States.

Understanding MS and how it affects the body is very challenging. MS is not a disease that plays fair. It takes unexpected turns at unexpected times. No one, who has been or is diagnosed, nor the most experienced MS specialist has definitely been able to predict the certainty of deprivation and deterioration of what any one person's MS may cause, or may not cause.

<u>JAMES 5:11</u> We give great honor to those who endure under suffering. Job is an example of a man who endured patiently.

III. MINI-AUTOBIOGRAPHY

The LORD is my Shepherd; I shall not want.
The LORD is my Shepherd; I have everything I need.
The LORD is my Shepherd; I shall not be in want.
Because the LORD is my Shepherd, I have everything I need.

    I was born, reared, and grew up in a small South Eastern Metropolitan town of Atlanta, Georgia.
    My immediate family included my father, my mother, two brothers, and two sisters. I was/am the youngest of my four siblings. I cherish the memories of the special years that I shared with my paternal and maternal families. Family visits, sleepovers, family reunions, and weekly gatherings, were just normal southern families functions. WOW!
    Although the many years spent with both sides of my grandfathers, I never knew or will know my true feelings of biological grandmothers. Ironically, both grandmothers had passed when I was born. However, I can vaguely remember my father's, father's (my grand father) second wife. Therefore, I did have a step-grandmother that I remember very little about.
    I grew up in a pre-dominant white majority segregated town. I remember Black/White town areas, home locations and communities,

sitting on the back of the buses, as well as "Blacks/Colored here and White only facilities. I went to the local movie theatre, where Blacks sat in the balcony, and Whites sat on the main floor. Can you imagine some of the advantages of those designated seats?

I attended a segregated school that housed grades one through twelve. Can you imagine being in a high school without a football team? Can you also imagine attending a school with elementary and high school sections in one building? Well, that is what I did. During that time, nothing negative was thought about the ages of the students. I, alone with other students, knew where I was supposed to be in the building. The population of the Black in the county was so small that everyone basically knew everyone else, as well as belonging to the limited family strands. Poor school behaviors were minute because the teachers, counselor, and the principal very often attended church with you. They very often shared dinners with students' families.

No, I did not grow up in a Utopia. I simply lived in somewhat of a protected vacuum where being segregated, poor, or deprived were not headlines news stories. Why? Because I have always been blessed to have practically everything I have ever wanted or needed. Remember, that I said practically everything I wanted. I did have everything that was necessary, and some choice items too.

I grew up with a father who worked, always had an automobile, a home, (even without plumbing for years, and that was common to every family), recreation, church, and a few dollars or cents in my pockets. My mother was basically a homemaker. I do mean a true and very creative homemaker. Varieties of food, clothing, hobbies, demanding daily chores, etc., were in abundance.

As for education, my Black segregated schoolteachers were tops and really knew how to teach. They knew their stuff. Think of this and compare learning/teaching with today's methods of teaching with modern technology heavily loaded in schools.

I attended one of the top four-year colleges in the pre-dominant Black Mecca of universities in the world. Just for information, there are also graduate schools among that predominant Black Mecca of higher learning institutions.

MULTIPLE SCLEROSIS, THE HORRENDOUS, NOTORIOUS, UNINVITED, INTRUDER

No brag, just fact, I never spent a day for make up in summer school doing college. I really had a good prior educational foundation. That credit goes to my prior teachers and my parents.

I chose a major in sociology and a minor in psychology. I had some very difficult subjects and professors. My college years were regular bondings with roommates, friends, and acquaintances from all areas. It was a full life college experience.

A month after college graduation, I married a neighborhood friend. During high school we were not boy/girl friends. However, we were always around each other, at school, on the bus, at church, functions held at his home, things held at my home, and nearly all other outings. Remember the small town factors.

We really never shared a typical boy/girl friend courtship while growing up. We were basically constant acquaintances. Most of our dating was through three years of mail correspondence across the miles from my college to his military station in Germany.

I became a military wife. It was a very unique learning and social experiences. I began to do social work for approximately the next two years. However, some few years later, after moving back to our home state, and becoming parents of two wonderful sons, I went to graduate school, acquired teaching credentials, and began to teach middle school for the next twenty-seven years.

In undergraduate school, never, ever, did I have any aspiration of teaching in anybody's school.

What happened? Well, after becoming a mother, and securing a house, one day I received a telephone call requesting me to become a substitute teacher. Today, I really still do not know who gave me the call. Remember small town again, where the educational head honchos knew that I was in town and possessed a teaching certificate. Any way, I gave the idea some thought. That would be an excellent way to be with my children and their schedules later on. That would also be a way to conserve my time and gasoline traveling twenty plus miles on the freeway daily, working in the social work or another field. Voila! I changed careers and really did enjoy it. My schedule was extremely compatible for transporting and attending my very active and busy sons' activities for more than two decades. My husband's schedule was conducive to the family's many activities and travels. Our working schedules worked well with individual and group activities schedules. Some times he took one son here, and I took the other son there, for various practices. Most of the times, we were able to attend their separate activities as one family.

We had some roller coaster years in our marriage. I have had a few thoughts that by statistics, we qualified to be a divorced marriage. Consequently, we struggled like the average couples in marriage. Sometimes, emotionally, physically, spiritually, and of course, sometimes financially.

However, through the magnificent Grace of GOD, we persevered.

We were, by America's standards, in the in-crowd sharing the American dream. Both of us had decent jobs. We had/have a large house/home in the suburbs, with a two car garage, two children, two dogs, a host of relatives and friends. We were very busy year round with activities, vacations, church attendance with participation, and material experiences. Fortunately, like every other family, we experienced some happy times and some sad times. We knew how to make adjustments.

I was truly blessed that the horrendous MS intruder did not show up until I was in my fifties.

My sons were grown. I had shared a very active life with them that would have been almost impossible with MS. Both were/are natural athletes and musical. Their school achievements and lifestyles, extra-curricula activities, and day-to-day endeavors were non-stop with things that we enjoyed with them to the highest. Providing finances for activities boosters, participating in travels, uniforms, and monetary necessities were somehow always supplied, plus some.

After one son's withdrawal from college, and then his completion of technical college life moved on. Then my other son's college graduation, and his marriage to my ex- beautiful daughter-in-law, by divorce. Fortunately, my ex-daughter-in-law and the family are in good friendly status with each other.

I have three biological grandchildren, and a slew of acquired grandchildren, and I do mean lots of loving acquired grandchildren through my husband and my acquaintances. We are with all of them very often on one accord, and with the different parents of all of the grands. I had begun to be in a very good comfort zone.

Basically, I have always been a healthy person. I worked and very rarely missed days or took sick leave. I too was an active person. I have achieved my career goals. Never, ever, did I want to become self employed and be my own boss. Back in the dark ages, when I was a social worker, I was the number one supervisor for a period. It was around that period of time, that I knew that being a boss was not my goal. Yes, I can manage and handle the responsibilities well; I simply just do not care to do so, I enjoy times spent with my family, especially the grand children's shenanigans and love, and my in-law family. We are always celebrating something. HURRAH! The majority of us, presently, four generations, reside in the original small, but a lot more populated now, in the same metropolitan area.

PHILLIPIANS 2:14
Do everything without complaining or arguing so that you may become as pure children of GOD.

E. C. McCOLLUM-FLANIGAN

IV. SOMETHING IS DEFINITELY WRONG

<u>ROMANS 12:12</u> Rejoice in hope, be patient in suffering, persevere in prayer.

Did I listen to my body, as I should have? Well, yes, no, and maybe so.

Months passed into almost a couple of years, enduring regular life style endeavors and activities. Then, I realized that I could not ignore the physical discomforts that I was experiencing.

Reality had set in big time. What is going on in this once physical and mental excellent body of mine? I had taken many and many physical examinations, to no avail, just waiting for some kind of diagnosis. I had tried many prescriptions, over-the-counter medications, herbs, vitamins, exercises, a little counseling, and other suggested helpful things. Several top board certified physicians who specialized in specific Central Nervous System fields had examined me.

I had kept abreast with my personal research as much as possible. I had prayed and prayed. Others had prayed and prayed continuously for me for GOD'S healing. (I did not lose the faith)

Yet, I was still at square one without clarity. Nothing was coming together to match or ease my complaints and miseries.

I definitely had to begun listening to my body. Okay, somebody HELP me! Something is very wrong! I had/have forgotten the exact time period when the severe tightness and numbness had become dominant maladies for me. It was around that time that I really began to get off-balanced and clumsy.

It did not make any difference what type of shoes were worn. It did not make any difference, even when I wore shoes or walked inside bare feet. I owned dozens of pairs of shoes with and without heels in various styles and colors. Of course, I had stopped even trying to wear shoes with heels, simply trying to improve my balance. That common sense strategy did not ease my feet miseries. I gave most of my heels away to others.

"Something is Definitely Wrong." Where is help? I got encouragement from others who knew what I was going through. They would help and complement me by saying something like, "You really are doing well and looking great." I needed to hear those encouraging complements. Presently, I still like to hear encouragement to help me sustain my positive character.

On my quick, mini down times, I would think about what was really going to happen to me in my off set health status. I did not want to speculate on the answer to that question. No, I was not in denial. I simply was not going to let that old horrible invisible MS enemy (later diagnosis) bring me down to nothing. Now, I might describe my disaster somewhat comparatively to Lower Manhattan's Twin Towers of the World Trade Center on 9/11/02. (Unknown invader catastrophic disaster)

After finally finding out what that horrendous something was, even though I did not know what was wrong with me, I was still trying to keep the faith. I try to live by GOD'S faithful principle. What principle? Sure, I had questions when I was not being told what I was experiencing. The principle that GOD is able to heal in HIS timing and HIS will will be done.

PSALM 55:22
Cast thy burden upon the LORD, and HE shall sustain thee. HE shall never suffer the righteous to be moved.

V. ENDURANCE FOR A DIAGNOSIS

COLOSSIANS 1:1
We also pray that you will be strengthened with HIS glorious power, so that you will have all the patience and endurance you need…

During the mid 1990's, I realized that I could not pop a prescribed pill to make me feel better. No prescribed medications I took, relieved the horrible feelings of heat and tightness in my feet. I began to get tired of trying to explain to everyone what was happening to me.

They knew that I was uncomfortable. They knew that I visited physicians regularly without receiving any type of diagnosis. However, my physicians were/are very caring and tops. I was daily-asked questions from caring people about my physical dilemma:

>Are you feeling okay today?
>What is wrong with you?
>What did the doctor say?
>Did the new medicine work?
>Why don't you take this (?) or that (?)?
>Why don't you just quit working and retire?
>Why don't you just take a Sabbatical and rest?

> Have you tried various herbs and holistic methods?
> Where is your faith in GOD?
> Well, you know that you reap what you sow...

Other curious and inquisitive questions and comments are stated in Chapter VIII.

Comments could go on and on. People were cordial and wanted to know, as I did. Frustratingly, I could not supply sufficient answers to the comments and questions. My sensitivity, and being unable to sufficiently relay answers to their inquiries, sometimes did put me in a silently defensive ignorant spot.

I had tried and I had done everything my neurologists had recommended. My physicians had not given me a definite diagnosis at that time, regardless of all of the tests I had taken, or the consultation discussions. My physicians had suspected Multiple Sclerosis, but due to my age and race, my family history, as well as the absence of dominant multiple plaques revealed from my Magnetic Resonance Imaging (MRI) in my brain and spinal cord, they were not one hundred per-cent positive of that MS diagnosis.

I trusted my physicians. I felt comfortable communicating with them. My husband's work insurance paid the bills along with each of my small co-pay visits. What was the problem? Has not science passed the tests with all of its researches, modern technology, and advances in coordinating fields to relate something?

Redundantly, I too had researched everything I could find in the medical references, computer web sites, and conversations with acquaintances who had friends and relatives with symptoms like mine. How long would I have to endure before finding out my diagnosis? What else could I do during the pending diagnosis stage? How long would I have to endure waiting for the most appropriate medications to help give me relief of the devious then, suspected diagnosis?

My main neurologist had told me that he wanted to perform a lumbar puncture to better diagnose my case. I was not timid about receiving the lumbar puncture. I had had two spinal blocks when my two sons were delivered by Cesarean Sections. Thus, with up-dated personal research and my neurologist explanation, I had no fear about receiving the injection. Nevertheless, during that period, I was receiving spinal vertebrae adjustments from an excellent Christian chiropractor. I went twice weekly for the adjustments. The chiropractor suggested to me that maybe I should not take the lumbar puncture at that time. He stated and visually pointed out to me from the x-ray of my spine what he would be adjusting. He did not see any damage associated with my spinal cord that could not be corrected with proper adjustments. He stated that with his bi-weekly spinal manipulations, my back should be properly aligned, which would eliminate the incorrect nerve pressures and messages going to my feet. That sounded like I was on the road to progress. I was glad to begin receiving progressive and favorable help with the problem, after suffering with it so long.

I faithfully went for the adjustments twice weekly. Finally, after about three months of the adjustments and manipulations, we agreed that I would take a break since I had not made any improvements. I did relax during his mini-counseling pep talks. Well, my bubble was burst again. How long would I be enduring this misery? I also realized that the chiropractor was unable to see the myelin damage from my x-rays. My neurologist could see the myelin damage from the previous MRI that I had horribly experienced taking.

After the sessions with the chiropractor culminated, I decided to have the lumbar puncture procedure performed. I worked a half-day. I then left my students with a substitute. I checked in the outpatient section of the local hospital. My neurologist performed the procedure. It did not take long. Of course, I was in the fetal position and remained as still as possible. He and the nurse talked quietly to me concerning my physical feelings during the process. My doctor showed me the long needle that he would be using to withdraw the spinal cord fluid. My doctor showed me what the withdrawn spinal cord fluid looked like in the tube. After the procedure, I remained in a hospital private room for four hours so that I could be monitored and observed following the procedure. During that waiting time, I had a late light lunch; I dosed catnap style, and watched television intermittently. Before I was told to dress to leave, my neurologist returned to my room to follow up on my condition before my dismissal.

A few days later, my neurologist called to tell me the results of the lumbar puncture test. He stated that, with all of the tests that I had taken, and with all of the pills that I had also taken without positive results, he would definitely now diagnose my case as multiple sclerosis. Well, at last I had a diagnosis. I was okay, because I still believed that once I knew what the problem was, then I would definitely feel better with the proper medication. I put the knowledge that I had acquired, regarding no known cause or cure for MS temporarily under the rug. I really felt that something positive would be happening for me very soon. Ignorant is bliss. No? I really anticipated having some relief from my miseries after a diagnosis was found.

Once again, my neurologist told me about the deteriorating factors of MS. Realistically, I thought, "Why me, with such a terminal chronic debilitating disease, after being a healthy person all my life? I had been thoroughly, physically examined by at least six specialists during that ordeal. I had followed their recommendations 24/7. Most of all, I continually praised GOD, JEHOVAH RAPHAL, for HIS goodness and mercy, for a healing. Through that long time of suffering, I was forgetting what normal feet, bladder, and bowel functions felt like. Yet, through JESUS CHRIST, my LORD and SAVIOR, I survived the 24/7 idiotic MS true game playing mess.

I continued teaching, walking around off balanced as well as surviving other dysfunctions.

Finally, with the diagnosis, I had to mentally get a grip and face the fact that, the very rude MS thing had silently and invisibly intruded, uninvited, of course, in, my body and was too much of an irrational, stubborn parasite to leave.

I knew and always know that I will continue to pray and ask GOD for patience and wait for HIS healing time. I do know that, "No weapon formed against me shall prosper." So, the enemy weapon must flee.

2nd TIMOTHY 1:17 For GOD has not given us the spirit of fear: but of power, And love, and have a sound mind.

VI. DIAGNOSIS AND CONSEQUENCES

PSALM 6:2 & 3
Have compassion on me, LORD for I am weak. Heal me LORD, for my body is in agony. I am sick at heart. How long, O LORD until YOU restore me?

After continuous physical examinations, after taking expensive medications without absolutely no physical relief, and trying not to fall apart emotionally for over two years, the multiple sclerosis diagnosis was given.

Was there any consolation for me knowing the long awaited diagnosis? Ironically, yes, and no, as I have shared bits and pieces to this saga earlier.

YES, in spite of all of the MS knowledge I had acquired, I truly felt that a diagnosis would give me the control that I needed to kick the intruder out. Finally, I could be prescribed medication that would relieve me of the invisible intruder's misery I lived with 24/7. I thought that the long agonizing testing period was finally over and specific help was on the way. However, after over two years of being questioned about my noticeable lessened demeanor, and after being examined by several top-notched board certified specialists, as well as my intense research, I still was not fully ready to accept that I had an incurable terminal disease. I still wanted to believe that once a diagnosis was positively identified, my prognosis would be medically controlled. (I knew, what had been the longevity of the diagnosis because all of my physicians were/are top-notched physicians? I tried to explain the real dilemma earlier. No, I would not attend any quacks.)

With daily advances in medical and modern technology, I still believed that it was highly impossible for a catastrophic disease of the 1900's, not to at least have something to relieve the constant agony. Yes, I was/ am aware that cures for many diseases have been pending for multiple decades.

My physician's were/are very honest and up front with me. Consultations with them were/are great. Never, had I thought that I would have something so debilitating. Did I think that I was too good for anything like this to happen to me? NO!

I was not surprised when my neurologists and immunologist, very cordially and professionally explained to me that very unfortunately, they had prescribed the medicines they felt would give me the best positive results. Since MS intrudes in the body, deteriorating tissues and organs, the most effective medications are intravenous injections and periodic physical therapy. (My experience of using these methods will be discussed in a later chapter.)

Yes, I could finally tell caring people what my problem was/is. Just think, relatives and friends also had known for about two years also that I was having problems. Yes, I had a lot of explaining to try to do too. Yes, the diagnosis really gave me positive and specific supplications to ask GOD to answer. I know that HE will and does every day!

NO, it put me in situations that had to be addressed for a permanent maintenance basis.

It made me realize that I must deal with reality and projected consequences. My constant intensive research on MS and unbiased conversations with my physicians had unknowingly prepared me on living with the unwanted MS enemy.

No, it made me face my limited mobile capabilities that were required in teaching middle school students. I was not happy to retire, because I had planned on working to the full required thirty year period.

Even today, with the massive behavior problems with students, over-work, and mediocre pay for teachers, if I had to presently choose, I would definitely choose continuing teaching daily instead of being handicapped, uncoordinated, and feeling physically horrible.

No, the MS diagnosis made me re-group my survival strategies. It made me go within myself and trust my GOD faithfully, because my strength must come from JESUS CHRIST, my LORD and SAVIOR.

The consequences started me on my way applying for permanent stabilizing prescriptions.

My beloved husband managed all of the red tape required by his company's medical insurance to pay eighty percent of the costs of the extremely expensive prescriptions.

I had to believe and not negatively think that, what was the point in all of the required paperwork, using the remaining twenty percent to be paid out of my disability retirement check, if all would be to no avail. No, I lamely thought that. No, I did or do not go there ignorantly for my rationalization.

1st PETER 3: 14

But even if you suffer for doing what is right, GOD will reward you for it. So don't be afraid and don't worry.

E. C. McCOLLUM-FLANIGAN

VII. MEDICAL DISABILITY RETIREMENT

JEREMIAH 29:11
For I know the plans I have for you, "Declares the LORD", plans to prosper you and not to harm you, plans to give you hope and a future.

When I was fifty years old, I had developed a bone spur on my 4th toe of my right foot. I had surgery because the spot was painful and irritating while wearing a shoe. The job of teaching middle school required standing, stooping, walking, and carrying equipments and materials, etc. at least and approximately seven hours per day per week. The surgery and recovery went great. Everything healed correctly and on schedule.

About a year later, I began to experience slight numbness in the front part of my right foot. I had it checked by my podiatrist. He could not find anything out of order, but suggested that maybe a little scar tissue was developing in the previous year's operative incision. That was checked by a second podiatrist. The second podiatrist found nothing out of order and recommended that I should see a neurosurgeon soon.

At that time I also smoked, less than a pack of cigarettes a day. I also drank about eight cups of coffee daily. Naturally, it was suggested to me that I must stop smoking and drinking so much caffeine. Quitting was extremely difficult. I did eventually quit both, because by that time, the hard to explain, unexpected and unexplainable tightness and numbness abnormality were now in both feet. I had begun to be off balance in just routine walking.

I knew that smoking and drinking caffeine were polluting my temple/body religiously. One bad habit was enhanced by the other one. Today, I only drink decaffeinated coffee every once in a while. Coffee drinking was not good without smoking cigarettes. The two were cause and effect for me, as well as I was co-dependant on both of those habits. After quitting and sacrificing, and going through withdrawals from both habits, I was so disappointed, not from quitting the habits, but my first podiatrists had stated that my foot (at that time) ailment was almost surely due to the excessive amounts of nicotine and caffeine causing physical irritations to the nerve endings and manifestations within my body. Well, after abstaining, seemed like I was getting worse. With hind sight, I now know that that was the MS enemy's sneaky aggravations. Coincidentally, I have not relapsed nor slipped back into the habits of smoking cigarettes nor drinking caffeine beverages.

For approximately the next two years, I spent a lot of time with two neurologists, a neurosurgeon, a rheumatoid immunologist tissue specialist, receiving bi-weekly spinal adjustments with a chiropractor, exercise with a physical therapist, and later a few sessions with an original Chinese acupuncturist. I appreciated him being up-front by telling me that he would be unable to help me much, because those ailments and deficiencies were from the Central Nervous System, and he did not want me to waste my money on false hopes with acupuncture techniques with such a severe disease.

I was told by my physicians that I have been prescribed almost all of the possible medications in pills that should have relieved those very miserable non-stop 24/7 enemy's miseries. My main neurologist stated to me that he was a little puzzled because my symptoms did not fit well enough with the regular profiles of any of the central nervous system's diseases. I also knew that with my age and race, it was a somewhat tough situation for diagnosing my problem. My neurologist stated that he had been in conferences with some of his colleague about the symptoms I was experiencing.

MULTIPLE SCLEROSIS, THE HORRENDOUS, NOTORIOUS, UNINVITED, INTRUDER

He referred me to one of the area's catastrophic hospital Central Nervous System's neurologist.

More and more blood tests were taken. My veins are small and floating, so locating them and sticking more than once, did not help me much. Presently, I have forgotten most of the names of the prescribed medications and blood tests I took seeking for a diagnosis.

My first magnetic resonance imaging, MRI, was a closed horrendous, carved in my mind, nerve racking experience. I was so vulnerable at the time of the MRI and ignorant of the exact procedure that the enemy had a field day with my mind. Later, on I have had three more MRI's of the brain, the thoracic area, and my lumbar area that really had me very fearful remembering the first devastating experience. My husband remained with me for encouragement and support on MRI's two and three.

Open MRI number four, I wanted to prove to myself that I could take one alone. I did just fine.

Presently, I know that the images from the closed MRI shows the pictures that physicians want to see for very detailed of my brain. I cringe when I know that the time will come to endure another closed MRI. Now, I know that I may take a sedative before the closed MRI to help my emotions.

Again, my neurologist said that the results were a little puzzling. Puzzling because the white degenerative plaques were not showing in great magnitude in my brain to diagnose any specific disease as chronic as MS. So, why and how, was/am I having those deficiencies, when my brain was/is not sending or receiving messages through my spinal cord to my feet, or other parts of my body for malfunctions.

By that time, I was definitely experiencing organ malfunctions. I was experiencing severe bladder and bowel malfunctions. My bladder began to get the urge and simply just let loose. My bowel had begun not to get the natural urge and would not naturally let loose. Stay tuned for embarrassing true experiences in two other chapters of this book.

I then saw more specialists. I made appointments with a urologist and a gastroenterologist.

Both physicians were nice, though, and concerned. Both prescribed medications. Both prescribed "out patient" tests in each field seeking true diagnosis. Both were conclusive that no type of surgery would eliminate the problems. Various medical procedures and prescriptions were given to me. One was given to help manage the incontinence problem. Another was given to help with the irritable syndrome problem.

Presently, both are daily routines that I must handle. Sometimes there are presently still a few embarrassing accidents. The intake of liquids might help with the bowel problem, but the added intake of liquids will aggravate the incontinence problem. What a catch twenty solution! Is there help with those problems anywhere and somehow? To me, those were definite requirements for a retirement.

In the course of conquering the enemy's strategies, I was given such tests as: a Doppler, Ear/Eye Evoke Potentials, Diabetes, Cholesterol, Cryptogram, Colon scanning, Optic nerve, lots and lots of blood drawings for various tests, and on and on and on.

Finally, I was given a lumbar puncture. It revealed that there were/are minute centimeters or something like that, of myelin missing and the withdrawn spinal fluid lead to the diagnosis of the MS monster. This was helpful for my almost two years of, "What did the doctor say", ordeal from family and friends. However, it was not much easier because then came the questions:

> What is that disease?
> What did you do to catch that disease?
> Who has it in your family?
> Is it contagious?
> Will you be able to continue working?
> Why are you in the bathroom so often?
> Why are you wobbling, stumbling, and tripping when you are walking?
> Can't you pick up your feet better than that?
> What can I help you with?
> Are you going to get better or get worse?
> How long can you live with it?

MULTIPLE SCLEROSIS, THE HORRENDOUS, NOTORIOUS, UNINVITED, INTRUDER

Well, trying to explain MS was/is a difficult task. I know that those constant questions asked of me were from really caring persons. They were not rude nor noisy persons. They cared for me and really wanted to know what was wrong with me. I appreciated their concerns. I just got frustrated because I was unable to give them answers to their or even my questions during that time.

At that time I was still working and driving my two miles back and forth. Very often, I would drive home in tears. At work I had begun to feel bad, not to mention having to think about not having accidents or falling. My co-workers and friends were so helpful to me. They knew enough about my personality and behavior that they too knew that I was not my usual strong self. I made it to the end of that school year.

During the short summer vacation, after twenty-seven years of teaching: two were very active regular substituting or supply, and twenty-five were contract middle school teaching.

Ironically, I had begun my first full time teaching assignment in the remodeled and refurbished one through twelve grades segregated school from decades ago that I had attended. Through the years, and by the time that I began teaching, it had become a highly populated integrated junior high school.

Continuing faithfully in prayer during the summer vacation, I prayed for mobility and strength, and to regain control of my bladder and bowels. I was definitely not ready to retire at that point. I really did like my job, the children that I taught yearly. I had liked all of my principals, my super co-workers and immediate team teachers, the parents, and school support personnel. Sure, in all of those years there had been lots of negative behaviors I did not like in my students, but I liked the students and disliked their poor demonstrated behaviors. Sure, there were lots and lots of late working days, studies, staff developments, meetings, conferences, disruptive students, parties and other socials, a few deaths of adults co-workers and students, over crowded classrooms, busy, busy, busy daily preparations of tasks for students' achievements on definite required curriculum skills. Contrary to what a lot of people think, a teacher does not sit, looking pretty behind a desk waiting to receive unearned checks during the holidays and summers.

I asked for GOD to give me an answer of what I should do. My summer days were getting shorter. Sure, I had signed my contract for another year, but I knew in my heart and mind that I probably would not be able to make it physically all day every day, and all day without positive medical aid. I had faced the fact that I would not be physically able to return for another year feeling as I had when I left before summer vacation. I had experienced some slightly scary stumbles, some falls, and of course, a few bladder and bowel accidents. Some general irritations and aggravations because I was not working with my usual full stamina. What a dilemma!

One morning, while lying on my couch, I recognized a breakthrough. I awoke from a brief nap, to realize to my surprise that I had not waken up in time to make it to the bathroom. That was it! I had wet my clothes during my sleep. Immediately, I accepted my predicament. I was so glad that I had been at home. I really knew the emotional and physical deficiencies that were happening to me without getting any better. My health had not improved over the brief summer. Yes, I shared this with my husband, knowing that I would receive his usual support. The next day I called my principal and apologized to him for waiting so close to the new school opening to resign.

Very fortunately, my principal and co-workers knew that I was having mobility trouble. My principal was extremely cordial. He gave me reference names and phone numbers to call and begin the retirement process. Luckily, I had ended my 25th year of teaching. That meant that I was able to qualify and retire with a medical disability without being penalized.

The process of submitting triple physicians' reports to two disability retirement departments, and more physical examinations took four months before I received my first disability retirement check. I managed fine because I was paid for an abundance of sick leave that I had not used while teaching. I had accumulated the maximum plus days of sick leave. Of course, an enormous amount of my sick leave pay was withdrawn for taxes by the Internal Revenue Service. Why? That's the government.

MULTIPLE SCLEROSIS, THE HORRENDOUS, NOTORIOUS, UNINVITED, INTRUDER

I called all of my team-mates and close co-workers to personally tell them of my resigning decision. About two months later I was honored with a Retirement Reception. Most members of my very immediate maternal family and my in-law family. some of my already retired friends, some friends that were still teaching, some former principals, and on and on with fellowship and gifts.

Just a short rewind now to show how off balanced I had become. One day I was in my yard, I fell and broke my ankle. I knew that I was falling, but I was unable to align myself to avoid twisting with my weight falling on my left foot. Can you believe that I did not have enough trouble with my foot to create more misery. Does this sound like something from Murphy's Law? I heard the crack when the ankle bone broke. Luckily, my husband was in the house. I wobbled and crawled to the door.

In the local hospital's emergency, my foot was x-rayed and temporarily cast. I later had a hard cast put on at my orthopedic office. I survived with the whole-leg and foot cast for almost seven weeks. I was still mobile with the cast along with using crutches or a cane for support. My family was jewels.

Adjusting to unemployment, seeing and hearing school buses by pass my house were not too heart-breaking because I definitely knew that I could not have been able to stand, walk, stoop, carry life science equipment, or even carry a lunch tray in such a humongous building while teaching and supervising children. I was/am okay with it.

I became an expert "Pittler". As a matter of fact, I received my PH D in "Pittling", with a 4.0 grade point average. I had full time to indulge in hobbies of reading, crocheting afghans, a litter exercising, driving to and from errands, a little visiting, weekly sessions of All Women's Bible Study Class, luncheons with my sisters, spending time with my darling biological and acquired grandchildren schools various programs in and out of state, hanging out with my husband on his off days, and just plain old goofing off.

Do I miss teaching? Yes, of course, after twenty-seven years. However, I only regret that the enemy again got away with its slight tricks that caused me to change my lifestyle. But, a good lop-sided rationale is, I was going to retire in five years anyway. No, I am only saying that. That is not a good rational for what the enemy is trying to accomplish. I know better, The enemy is not going to take away most of my livelihood. Old enemy of MS, you have failed big time!

2nd CORINTHIAN 12:9

My grace is sufficient for you, for power is made perfect in weakness.

VIII. EMERGENCY HOSPITALIZATION

2ND CORINTHIANS 9: 8

And GOD is able to make all grace abound to you, so that all things at all times, having all that you will need, will abound in every good work.

    A few months after retirement, I had gotten the hang of using my cane (after the broken ankle predicament) when I was away from home. Members of my family also helped me carry items, such as purchased things in bags, food trays when dining in buffet restaurants, in stead of a waitress carrying them. They were great!

    Okay, one Sunday, I fell in my kitchen in front of the refrigerator. I tried to hold on to the adjacent counter to help me lift myself off the floor. I was unable to do so. I was alone, so I crawled to a nearby chair. I rested a few minutes, then I tried to walk to a near by couch. I did not make it, I fell again. At that time tumbling and falling did not upset me because, stumbling and loosing my balance were things that I very regularly experienced.

    As I tried to up lift myself again by boosting up my body with my hands, on the nearby couch, I was unable to do so. After several efforts, and very slowly moving upward, I was able to sit on the couch.

Maybe an hour passed and my husband arrived from work. He had gone outside, then I was able to go slowly outside after I had recuperated on the couch. Upon returning slowly in the house, I continued to sit. Some short time later, I thought that I would change clothes for bed. I was unable to climb seven steps independently. Between my husband and myself, I made it upstairs to my upstairs' bedroom. I had no idea what a true exasperation was until then. I remembered my physicians questions concerning when had I had a last attack.

I was put to bed by my husband. GOD made it easy for me that night. The next morning I realized that I had slept well. I was very proud of myself for not having to use the bathroom, and not be able to get to the bathroom during the night. Prior to this major incident, I had gotten use to arising at least once during the night to use the bathroom.

When I awoke the next morning, I also tried to get out of bed like usual. I could not. Again my husband had to help me to the bathroom to also take a sponge bath and get dressed in clothes I had asked him to get for me. Lending and holding onto him, I managed to get dressed.

I then called my neurologist who worked at the metropolitan catastrophic hospital with the MS unit. Unfortunately, I nor my husband were able to connect with him so that I would know what to do. After being transferred to several in-hospital numbers and being left on hold, I decided to call my local neurologist. He had/has always been speedy and dependable in returning calls. However, I had not called him first because I had thought that since my metro neurologist directly practiced where I thought I needed to be for an immediate emergency, that my metro neurologist was the one that I needed to contact. Fortunately, my local neurologist returned my call immediately and told my husband and I the specific procedures to follow.

Coincidently, my younger son and his four year old daughter were temporarily vacationing with us from out of state. I had planned on closely nurturing and spending the whole week pampering my young and loving granddaughter.

MULTIPLE SCLEROSIS, THE HORRENDOUS, NOTORIOUS, UNINVITED, INTRUDER

After their vacation with us, my husband and I had completed plans to be on a scheduled seven day cruise in the Western Carribbean.

My thoughts were becoming haggard. How would I be able to share that planned time with my family, my granddaughter, and enjoy a seven day cruise, when I was unable to get myself around?

Time was passing and I was unable to rise and stand up from my seat. My husband and son picked me up and put me in the vehicle. I simply told my granddaughter that I truly loved her and that I had to go to the doctor because I was unable to walk at that time. She was sweet, kissed and hugged me. She was fine because she was with her daddy.

The hospital was about a forty minute drive. Arriving at the adjacent admission hospital, I was met by a medical personnel with a wheelchair. My local neurologist had called for my entrance. I spent about five hours going through paperwork and physical preliminaries. I had been a hospital patient on occasions for other ailments before, but I did not know what to expect because this was a whole new circumstance for me.

Luckily, it was my husband's off day from work. He patiently sat in the examining room with me throughout the rest of the day. We were there long enough to be served lunch. He also patiently stayed with me most of the night after my transfer to the Spinal Catastrophic Hospital.

Nurses wheeled me to take a foot x-ray (checking to up-date on my previous broken ankle). I took various blood tests. I answered lots of medical and insurance questions for my triage medical history. The nurses and technicians were cordial. I had to be adjusted in the bed to use the bed pan.

After a while, it was explained to us that my neurologist wanted me to be admitted to the somewhat adjoining CNS Catastrophic Hospital. Then I was met by a nurse from there and wheeled through the connecting hospital's decorative painted tunnel.

I knew a little about that hospital by living in the metro area. I knew that it was one of the best of its type in the country for paralyzed and comatose patients. I had taught the brother of one of its critically damaged young patients who had become dominantly paralyzed from playing and falling out of a tree.

Being pushed in the wheelchair, I did not see any patients walking in the corridors as I have always seen in other hospitals while visiting or when I was a patient. By that time, it was night. I had to wait outside of the room I had been assigned too while the other patient was being seen by her physician or nurse.

Briefly waiting outside of the room in semi-darkness, my emotions began to become questionable. Remember, I had spent hours not knowing what was going on. Just sitting in that wheel chair began to make me think negatively about not being able to walk again.

I was soon wheeled into the room. The dividing privacy curtain was closed so I was unable to see the other patient. Well, as I was put in the bed, there was an opening in the curtain wide enough for me to see my roommate. I introduced myself and my husband to her and fell apart. I shed many crocodile tears and complained to her about my very long day and that I could not walk.

She told my husband and me her name. She asked me if I would mind if the privacy dividing curtain stayed open. Of course, that's really what I wanted to happen too. Even though my bed was next to the window, I was too glad to keep the curtain opened all of the following stay, unless the staff was performing some personal hygiene tasks.

Throughout my selfish crying and pity pot episode, I heard her testimony. She told me that I was so blessed and that everything would work out fine. I immediately recognized that GOD had made this meeting and sent her to be my personal angel. I fail to express how gracious and thankful I was/am to have met such a compassionate and caring person at the peak of my being so vulnerable.

She shared with me that she had been hospitalized, remaining in bed without sitting out of bed, or without being wheel chaired any where for nine months straight. Her only moving activity included required "turn the body over" positions, periodically daily and nightly by the nurses.

MULTIPLE SCLEROSIS, THE HORRENDOUS, NOTORIOUS, UNINVITED, INTRUDER

For some time, I do not remember exactly how long now, she had also been in another hospital for months. She had then been transferred to the specialty hospital for the last nine months. In spite of all of her permanent disabilities, she appeared to be an excellent "happy camper."

She was diabetic, her left leg had been amputated above the knee, she wore a permanent catheter, she wore a permanent colostomy bag, her vision was severely blurred even wearing corrective lens glasses, she was quite overweight, and she had some heart and lungs damages which required her to periodically breathe pure oxygen through temporary attached apparatus. Above all, to me, she had the born again heart of gold and continuous encouraging words of an angel.

She assured me that I was going to be alright. She told me that she was very glad that I did not mind opening the dividing personal area curtain. She stated that she was very happy to share the room with me, especially because she had resided in that particular hospital for months, and all of her former roommates did not want the privacy curtain opened. WOW! She could finally see on the other side of the room, look out of the window, and have conversation with people beside the staff members and members of her family when they visited. I really felt good hearing her share with me. I felt like I was a little part of helping somebody as I passed prayfully along to walking mobility.

My prior hospital stays had been in well selected private rooms. I had requested the privacy because I was comfortable and peaceful that way. My quests did not have to disturb a roommate and visa-versa. I am sure that I had probably requested a private room at the catastrophic hospital too, but, remember I had waited at least a half of day for availability of admission.

I am also positive that GOD knew that I would need specific companionship during that devastating physical and emotional ordeal. I was a wretch for a while there. My words come short of truly expressing my actual emotional up-lifting after communicating with my beloved roommate.

I had been hospitalized on a few other occasions. I had undergone two Caesarean sections, a complete hysterectomy, (fibroid tumors) foot surgeries, left breast benign biopsy, etc. Okay, I know that you might be thinking, "I thought that the author stated earlier that she had been healthy before the intruder's disruption? Well, do you know what? You are correct! To me and according to female statistics and actual positive female admittances, the fore stated surgeries are very common and correctable. Therefore, I was healthy because undergoing those surgeries were pieces of cake and very common.

Presently, I think that because the majority of females nation wide, have probably had, or will probably have, some, all, or some other comparable female common surgery, that I was healthy. I say that because those surgeries are ones with positive prognoses, then patients quickly move on.

Any way, back to my roommate and our compatibilities. During our initial conversation, after my husband had left to go home, she and I talked throughout the night, intermingled between the nurses' visits checking both of us. Well, it was wonderful conversation. We were not intruding on each others private sleep time, because we knew that we would not have to get up early to go anywhere. Our open shared communication revealed that we had some things in common.

Comparatively, she had taught special education in a middle school for years prior to her failing health. Presently, I cannot remember how many years she told me she had taught. She had two adult sons. One of her sons had a shaky marriage. The other son worked, but did not manage his finances well. In spite of her long-termed disability and long convalescence, her sons were constantly depending on her for financial support. Her married son, his wife and two children lived in her house paying very little or very limited amounts for his family's maintenance and security. By the way, she wrote their/her monthly bills during the period that I shared a room with her. I met her married son, his wife, and their two children. She met my sons and my precious granddaughter while visiting also. A sad part, I guess, was that her husband had left her when her health began to fail. I think that I am remembering it correctly. That hurt me to hear her share that because she was such a loving person to me. What type of love and support is there when your spouse or significant other walks out when you need them the most? I know, I know, and I still know that marriage relationships, or whatever, are two-sided situations. However, I did not hear the whole two-sided story. I negatively acquired an attitude about her ex-husband whom I did not meet. I knew positively well that was the wrong judgmental and prejudice thing to do. I did not know their prior ups and downs or their lifestyles. But, at that time, I thought, "How did that happen to such a sweet and caring person"? I did not know what had gone wrong between them. We shared a lot of things, but we did not share our intimate positive and negative marriage truths.

She was so positive with my visitors. Even today when we periodically communicate by telephone, she always sends greetings to my immediate family members. I return the same greetings to her family. My husband and I with two of the grandchildren have visited her in her hometown hospital.

It was an extraordinary good visit and reunion for all of us.

My first days in the hospital, I was pumped up big time with injections of intravenous steroids. The dosages of the beneficial steroids elevated my blood pressure high as a kite. The high blood pressure was treated and it returned to normal. The steroids side effect kept me blabbing non-stop to everyone who came in the room. I do not remember some of the things I said, or to whom I said the things too. I do remember saying good things to everyone about my roommate.

When my Pastor visited, I requested that he would say a prayer with her too. My Pastor would have done it anyway without my request.

One of the main purposes of that amount of steroid injections was to relax my nerves in the central and the peripheral nervous systems. In order for my body's systems to coordinate again, my nervous systems had to be relaxed and enlightened as much as possible in a shorten time period as possible.

I was introduced to an in-house multiple sclerosis specialist. He was my daily neurologist while I was hospitalized. I was introduced to an in-patient case worker, several personal attending nurses, and medical technicians. I was assigned to a male plus a female physical therapists.

I was wheeled to very beneficial MS and care-giver counselor sessions covering topics from A to Z on ways to manage MS as well as not wearing one's caregiver down.

After staying in bed and completing the prescribed dosages of the steroids, I began going to intensive physical therapist in the gymnasium area. Initially, after breakfast, receiving medications, personal hygiene, and dressing, with the assistance of my female therapist, then I was wheeled to the gym on my floor for physical therapy (PT).

I did acclimate comfortably to my surroundings in a few days. I had so many choices and so much food served that I always saved some for my husband's after work nightly visits.

With my shattered thoughts of, "What's going to happen to me" state of mind and temporary insecure emotions, I witnessed first hand the conniving thief's obvious effects it had stolen from patients.

Sitting in my wheel chair in the gym, my initial sight of the conditions of the patients I saw, is a permanently carved in stone mental image.

There were approximately thirty patients in my gym area. They/we were very well supervised by therapists, nurses, and counselors. Patients were in wheelchairs on exercise mats and tables. Patients were being assisted by individual caregivers on various types of exercise/therapy equipments.

I heard only one patient conversing with a therapist.

My therapist briefly explained an overview of what I was observing as well as the strategies and purposes of the skills that I would begin trying to regain. I heard my therapist. I wanted to believe my therapist, but at that eye-opening observation, as I not only watched patients' necks, hands, feet, and parts of their bodies be manually assisted by the therapists, to be exercised, because they had lost control of moving their bodies appendages. The reality thoughts that came to me were, "This is it for me. I was going to be a burden to someone the rest of my life. No, I refuse to become a vegetable."

At that initial session I also thought that like those patients, I would be permanently wheel chair bound. I was not ready to accept that I would become a permanent 24/7 disabled dependant to anyone. I knew that my house was/is tri-leveled, without a bathroom on the main floor. My husband work shifts were all kinds of hours, sometimes days and sometime nights. How would I be able to take care of myself without a constant caregiver? My husband would help, but it would be impossible for him to work full time, take care of the house, shop, cook, attend to his personal health needs, take care of me full time, including my regular visits to physicians, attend church, and have some relaxing time and friendship time for himself.

Sure, I had/have plenty of family members living very near by me. It was very frustrating when I thought that I would have to depend on anyone completely to take care of me for the rest of my life.

I knew from naturally observing and being around handicapped relatives, persons in stores, churches, amusement parks, special needs and impaired students, and some of everybody and everywhere with mental or physical disabilities lived and survived with struggles.

I sat in my wheel chair observing others to help me become acclimated to my peers and some of the routines that patients endured striving for success. I observed patients that were assisted from wheel chairs to crutches and walkers. I observed patients that were assisted from wheelchairs on types of slim boards, then slowly, and what appeared to be painful slide with assistants' help on exercise mats and tables. I saw patients whose fingers and toes had to be manipulated with help for exercising.

Thus, the caregivers were quietly speaking to their patients as they assisted them. Also, remember that was/is a very special Central Nervous System Catastrophic Hospital where like me, the in-house patients were unable to walk and many could not talk.

The uniform dress-code and standard equipment for patients were wheel chairs where every patient had an attached catheter bag or wore adult diapers. A few patients had portable oxygen canisters attached. Some patients wore loose fitting sweat suit like clothing during therapy sessions, including me. Some patients wore special hospital like gowns all of the time. Nurses and therapists were always available to get and return patients to their rooms to change patients' clothes in cases of bladder and bowel accidents.

One day after I had been hospitalized for about a week, I was on an exercise matted table being aided by my therapist during leg bends, I had a bowel accident. I was not embarrassed, even though I did apologize to him. My therapist aided me in getting in my wheel chair, so that I would be able to go to my room, clean and change myself. Then I would return to therapy, only if I wanted to complete the interrupted session. I had worn a pair of dark sweat pants. My female therapist helped me with my baths, personal hygiene, personal counseling when needed, made sure daily that I wore an adult diaper along with the catheter. No, I was not embarrassed at that time because I had personally experienced and seen other patients experience slips. It was not an uncommon thing to happen there. Remember, patients had lost body functions controls. Loosing functional body controls were common place there.

I along with other patients, males and females, had received a very good and speedy education on the serious problems and ways of handling bladder and bowel problems due to the lack of destroyed Central Nervous System brain transmissions messages going to and from the brain with CNS impairments. Considerations and explanations were very common in the Bladder, Bowel, and Skin Programs.

Like any type of institution, the faster one adjusts to the circumstances and accept the reality of what happens, the faster and content a person will be adjusted to any particular program.

My very kind and compassionate roommate always had comforting words for me when I experienced new and different survival styles of living. Because we always kept the dividing curtains opened, except during personal examinations by individual nurses and physicians, I shared mostly everything about my debilitating health. I cried, she comforted me from her bed.

There were times that I did feel sad for her. I got that feeling as I was able to independently transfer from my bed to my wheel chair and wheel chair myself out of the room to attend physical therapy sessions or just leave the room to goof off quickly in the halls.

During visits with my family members, they would wheel me to other areas, inside and outside of the hospital. There was my new found friend who appeared content and spiritual, and who had not been out of bed for many months. Not to mention that she had naturally missed seeing GOD'S beautiful and natural creations. (sun, moon, grass, rain, clouds, etc.)

How could I put my problems on her back? She was just that type of GOD-given person who helped me confront and bare the things that had changed in my life. GOD had performed a miracle to me through her. I did not feel guilty when I thought that maybe I was too over-bearing to her with my discomforts. However, several times I did think and ask her, "What have I done for you lately?" She always responded with such positive loving replies.

Momentarily, I am rewinding back to my initial entrance in the physical therapy area of the particular floor that I occupied. There were several floors for intensive patients' residences who had CNS damages. It was/is a big hospital.

In my group there were a few teen-agers through senior citizens aged patients. There were about the equal number of males and females. There were about the equal number of Blacks and Whites. (I do not recall my views of other ethnic groups. CNS patients were there or somewhere being treated I pray.)

A real eye-opener that really filled me with GOD'S gratitude to me was, when I first witnessed a few patients who were unable to control the movements of opening and closing their lips. Caregivers/caretakers had to manually open their lips in other to guide straws into their mouths for them to sip liquids. I later found out that the hospital also housed patients who had to take liquids and nourishments through intravenous methods.

Can you believe that I had cried and complained about the inability to walk? Yes, I had, and occasionally I do. Are there just comparisons? Minor problems are major problems to some of us.

I saw patients who had to be hooked with straps and coordinating apparatuses in order to be mechanically hoisted onto and off the therapy tables. Never, had I imagined a sight like that. Human beings hoisted to and from therapy tables in order to receive as much help as possible in order to survive. How great GOD is to me! However, that was/is great because the immobile patients are still able to receive some treatments.

I heard a male patient talking with the therapist. The voice got my attention because most other patients were silent. For a day or two I watched this young male patient seriously struggling, with the aid of his therapist, trying and succeeding, what appeared to be painful and aggravating, using a special wooden apparatus to transfer from his wheel chair to an exercise/therapy table. Again, he was one to the two patients that I had heard speaking. I had witnessed the caregiver helping him drink liquids by using straws, after positing his lips in a specific position.

Luckily, somehow, at some time, we introduced ourselves to each other. We intermingled communicated with each other and our therapists. We exchanged verbal and mini-autobiographies with each other. Our therapy tables were near each other because we shared the same two therapists.

He was married and had small children He shared a good life with his family. He and his family lived in the neighboring metro county where I resided. He enjoyed many activities and was an active sportsman. He was a computer employee. In short, he had taken a flue shot. I do not remember if that was the first flue shot that he had taken. He told me that three days after receiving the flue injection, he had become approximately ninety percent paralyzed. He was able to only partially control his head, neck, his hands, arms, and his legs and feet in very limited positions.

No, I am not speaking negatively about flue injections. I am unaware of all of the detrimental facts and medical history of his case to be negative. I do not qualify to be judgmental about what went wrong.

I witnessed him having excellent positive determination that he was going to overcome that paralysis and regain his mobility in a short time. He had been hospitalized for rehabilitation and extensive therapy for several months.

I was happy to share conversations with someone in therapy besides my caregivers. My husband and other visitors visited me between or after my PT sessions. It was very consoling to hear how another person had really been brought down and was positive and inspiring enough to know that he would get back up in GOD'S timing.

The other person that I heard talking was an older teenager who had been shot in or near the medulla area in connection with a gang fight. I do not know how long he had been in rehabilitation, or what his expected prognosis was to be. He would stand up from his wheel chair by using crutches. I do remember him awfully walking around with the crutches. I also heard him conversing with another young fellow and his therapist.

Later, when I had moved to another level during my rehabilitation, one day while walking in the hall using a three/four wheeled walker, and assisted by my therapist who fastened a safety belt encircling my waist and extending to him, so that I (and other patients) would be secure avoiding stumbles and falls. I inquired to my therapist about the situations of patients in closed rooms and patients on the other floors of the hospital. I was informed that because that was an extraordinary specialty hospital for patients with critical Central and Peripheral Nervous Systems dysfunctions, there was a section of the hospital that housed exclusively comatose patients as well as patients who had become human vegetables as well as other brain impaired patients. Not only did the hospital provide bedding for the patients, the hospital also provided temporary housing accommodating intermittently for the patients immediate family members. Those accommodations were basically within walking distances if necessary, from the hospital. Some business corporations also helped to financially provide that most needed housing services for the immediate family members.

Often times, my husband would wheel me outside of the hospital to a seating area. One day I was able to lift myself out of my wheelchair by holding and lifting myself onto the outside bench, all by myself. There was/is an outside sitting area near the emergency ambulance patients' admission entrance. There I witnessed many incoming patients from the very young to senior citizen ages. I could hear attendants conversations concerning some of the local and long distances the patients had traveled to be admitted to the hospital. Some of the patients had come with medical attendants and possibly one or two close family members, from out of state in emergency vehicles and ambulances.

Admission to that hospital was the best one for them to receive the extraordinary brain care that would be needed for their medical improvements.

Other in-house patients, as myself were rolled outside to take in some fresh air. On a couple of occasions I saw some of the in-house patients lifted in their wheelchairs by automatic ramps and lifts in medical vehicles. Then they were rolled in specific spaces in the vehicle where the wheelchairs were locked in place to keep them from rolling while being transported. The patients were also hooked with special seat belts to make sure that each patient was enclosed in the wheelchair in its special area to keep the patients from falling out of the chairs. Of course, there were enough medical chaperones accompanying them.

With proper assistance from the caregivers, the special medical vans/buses would take specific able groups on various field trips to professional sports games, sightseeing in the city, museums and other cultural and recreational outings. Most of those patients had been assigned in the hospital for a while.

Finally, after sixteen days of daily hours of intensive physical therapy, I was able to walk in the halls, and up and down stairs using the guard rails and a cane., along with the direct belting with my therapist. I had progressed from the wheelchair and the special walker only with proper supervision. Thus, I still had to use the wheelchair for required security. Frankly, I was walking with assistance of a prop, but I was still unsteady and off balanced without a prop.

Presently, I use my cane practically everywhere except in my home. In my home I am able to hold onto pieces of furniture and stair rails. Yes, I do fall on a daily basis all of the time. I have lots of physical and ugly scars, but I get around independently. God helps me up. I thank JESUS CHRIST, my LORD and SAVIOR daily for my mobility. I could not walk, jump, run, squat, or spin on a dime too independently, but Praise goes to GOD that I am able to move from place to place without a wheelchair. HALLELUJAH to HIS name! I am able and very regularly drive in bumper to bumper free-way traffic. To me, my parallel parking is better than it has ever been.

MULTIPLE SCLEROSIS, THE HORRENDOUS, NOTORIOUS, UNINVITED, INTRUDER

My physician explained to my husband and I that even though most patients remained in that hospital for months, I was an exception and I was at a stage that I could be dismissed from the hospital if I was mentally ready, and would have some assistance in my home when needed.

I was so elated that I cried big time again at the news. I wanted to go home. However, I experienced a real emotional down. There I had been admitted and ready to be dismissed, and what was my problem? Of course, I was really happy with the exit news. WOW!

I was getting ready to be dismissed and I had to purchase, with my husband's insurance and my out of pocket money, several pieces of required maintenance equipment. One of the main key beneficial philosophies of the hospital was/is to be prepared for the worst situations that could happen. Tough!

Thus, I left the hospital with an order for an expensive wheel chair that the thick cushion had been measured and customized for my legs, back, and hips measurements. I left the hospital with a very durable potty-chair, a three/four wheel walking cart with a folded pull out seat attached, and a professional shower bath chair. I had experienced hands on training on how to use each piece of the equipment properly from my therapists.

At that time. my supportive and beloved husband handled all of the insurance requirements, as well as supplying the man-power along with my male therapist that was necessary in getting the items and putting them in our vehicle for transporting them home.

As the final dismissal pieces of the process were put together to make things better for me as that old devious intruder played havoc with my physical circumstances, I had another mind boggling reality that I had to accept. I was extremely disappointed when I had to face the fact that I had to keep a catheter connected and attached. I guess I had chosen not to hear that earlier. I had thought that the catheter would be removed before dismissal.

My physician and nurse had explained to me that it was very important to keep the catheter connected in order to be sure that my female organ skin did not stay wet. For some strange reason that I had failed to clock in, during my hospital stay my attached catheter bag had to be emptied often by my nurse. So, I was urinating a lot, from the medication side effect. There was another way of managing urine called an IC. I had not been trained for that method, and by my somewhat early dismissal, there was not enough time for that particular training.

There I was ready to go home and would have to walk around with a "pee" bag hanging around my ankle. I was told that I would probably have to wear the catheter for maybe one or two weeks. Then I should return to the hospital's out-patient section for a check-up Thank GOD, my husband had paid attention to instructions on how to change the day catheter to the bedtime catheter. I paid very little attention at all. I am also glad that he paid attention on the preparation of my daily medications and the proper procedure for my daily injection. I was ready to leave with bag and baggage. My husband had packed flowers and gifts that I had received during my stay. I patiently kissed, hugged, and told my roommate goodbye. I gave her one of my flowers too. We knew that we would keep in touch through phone and by mail. We shared the same telephone three free prefix numbers.

Okay, I got my act together. I put on a pair of black sweat pants with an ankle zipper to hide the catheter. Surprisingly, for some strange reason, at that most needed time, the zipper broke. "Boo hoo, boo hoo", and more sobbing. Luckily, I was going home and I would not have to be seen by anyone.

That worked, I did not see anyone. My older son lived in the metro in an apartment. My younger son and his daughter had returned to their home state. I talked to a few people on the telephone. I told my husband that I cared not to receive quests. He did/does understand. He changed my day/night catheter bag, prepared and injected my medications that night and the next morning.

At some point, early the next day, my light bulb went on full wattage to make an appointment with my local urologist. Bingo! I could go the next day. Now, I had to see how well I could drive, or find a driver to chauffer me. I went on a short drive with my husband. I did great after my husband got home from work. The family two close family members that I had asked, unknowingly had made unbreakable important plans because they did not know that I would be at home.

MULTIPLE SCLEROSIS, THE HORRENDOUS, NOTORIOUS, UNINVITED, INTRUDER

I told my husband that I really wanted to drive the five miles to the urologist. Since I had been so distraught at the hospital, I did not know what I would feel like if I had to continue walking around with the exposed catheter. How would I explain that to my small relatives and grandchildren? Farther more, not all adults would understand the situation either.

Well, I had lost bladder urgent stoppage control. That horrible, sly, and unwanted intruder had sneaked in and robbed me of that control. I would probably have to wear the adult diaper and underpants.

The next day my caring husband informed me that he was going to get off work near my appointment time to go with me to the urologist. He lovingly stated that he did not want me to be alone, especially if the news would be negative and I had to keep the catheter attached.

Can you beat that?

I was thrilled that he would be accompanying me because I did not know what prognosis my urologist would tell me. My husband knew the emotional turmoil I had gone through when I was told that I would need to wear it a while for my protection and hygiene. So he stood by me.

I prayed for the removal of the catheter. I can truly praise and thank GOD for answering my supplication immediately. During the appointment, after the nurse had disconnected the catheter, I left a specimen to be examined. I was given some type of cytology urinary tract ultra sound. I urinated naturally to see that the normal release of urine was naturally passable since a catheter had been attached for a while. VOILA! I passed everything. I was so relieved that I would be able to come and go without explaining and being questioned by others. PRAISE GOD!

The after effect was realizing that the horrendous unwanted pest had robbed me of a normal, bladder, kidney function. Through continuous trials, errors, and accidents, I adjusted to reality.

The bladder problem was not going away, due to the MS intruder, even by taking retention bladder medication daily! Therefore, I must be strategic and beat the intruder's game play.

Well, the horrific intruder played its game on me. I have learned to watch my fluid intake, especially the days that I am going to be away from my home.

Basically, wherever I go, I find the location of the nearest restroom before I get settled too comfortably. The support of my family, the attentiveness of hospital physicians, staff, and all caregivers, gave me just what I needed to restore my mind and mobility.

My roommate was attributed to my spiritual and emotional stability. I sincerely thank and praise JESUS for letting an angel come into my life when I needed one the most. The hospital staff clergyman did visit me following up from an admission inquiry if I would like to be visited by the clergy. Yes, my personal pastor was extremely consoling on his visit, as he always is.

Today, I go to the same hospital about three times a year for the MS out-patient continuous checkup and prescriptions refills. I am kept up to date on seminars magazines, MS monthly Group meetings and testimonies, National MS Society news, teleconferences, MS Family Fun Functions, etc, with family members. My experience with the health professionals, other patients, and the whole over-all help have really helped me to be the surviving person that I am today and forever.

1ˢᵗ PETER 5: 6 &7

6) Humble yourselves therefore under the mighty hand of GOD, that He may exalt you in due time: 7) Casting all you care upon Him; for HE careth for you.

IX. PHYSICAL STRENGTHS AND WEAKNESSES

JAMES 5:13
Are any among you suffering? Keep on praying about it. Those who have reason to be thankful should continually sing praises to the LORD.

How can one be strong and during the same period be weak? How can one be positive and during the same period be negative? How can one be independently blessed, and yet be dependent? The answers yes to these questions depicts a lot of truths when one lives with a terminal illness.

In reference to the previous chapters' denotations concerning my physical health profile, basically, I had been in good health. As stated in an earlier chapter, I had gone "under the knife". several times. All of those surgeries culminated with excellent results. I had/have been very conscientious in routinely maintaining my dental and my vision in super conditions.

Ironically, again, how can I state that I was in good health, when I had undergone those health deficiencies? Well, based on statistics documented from physicians, medical records, and standards, I had common ailments that were medically and physically successfully repairable.

Praise GOD! There was always lights in the tunnels for those prognoses. I had never been overweight or a physically inactive person. I was not a daily exerciser, but I walked, jogged, ran, swam, bowled, danced, minimal aerobics, and other non-strenuous physical activities throughout my life. I just did not always do them routinely.

Today, I keep physically active by cautiously walking short distances using my cane, and using a shopping cart as support when store browsing. I try to ride one or two miles on my stationery bike, walk about one or two miles on my treadmill. I also participate in aquatic exercises and periodic physician prescribed physical therapy sessions. However, I admit that I fail to do those exercises daily many times. Why? My personal choice to be lazy. I choose to rationalize and participate as I want to do so.

I am blessed to be able to drive my regular vehicle in freeway and bumper to bumper traffic.

I am truly blessed that my hands have super dexterity. I have to concentrate on my feet movements while moving around, but I refuse to allow the MS intruder any breaks in keeping me from coming and going where I please. I simply out smart the sneaky idiot. I listen to my body. When I need to rest a few minutes to regroup my strength, I do so.

I am extremely grateful to be so mobile, in spite of being slow and clumsy. How does it feel to pivot to catch or throw an object? Just think, what fun it is to run up and down stairs? Presently, I do not know, but I can certainly cherish those experiences and memories. Yes, I am in control. I am steadily on the move. I fall frequently somewhere, usually around my home, and my GOD lets me get up!

My physical disabilities really can make some things difficult. But, I am beating the MS enemy at its own game. I change the rules better than it does. I have almost forgotten how the feel of normal feet and lower legs are suppose to be. I have almost forgotten the normal feelings of being able to hold urine until I decide to relieve it. How does it feel to have a regular bowel movement at a regular time? How does it feel to take a nap during the day or night?

MULTIPLE SCLEROSIS, THE HORRENDOUS, NOTORIOUS,
UNINVITED, INTRUDER

Low emotional swings aggravate the physical and vice versa. Many times as stated earlier, it has really been easier not to be truly candid about how I felt/feel, than it was/is to respond to family and acquaintances, when they inquire about my health. Simply, when someone asks, "How are you?" Sometimes, it is easier to respond by lying and saying, "I am super and just fine," rather than saying, "I feel completely miserable and horrible." My feet feel miserable and abnormally tight. My walking is always off balanced and wobbly. But it is still harder to try to explain my adequate miserable malady, than to lie and say, just fine.

I have observed and accepted the nerve damage skin appearance. In certain areas, the skin appears as though my skin is suffering from some degree of burn injury. One day I really looked at my hands. They looked rough, as though I had been doing some rigorous out door manual labor. I really examined the darkened parts of my knuckles. They resembled the knuckles of a gorilla.(?) I knew the answer to that cause and effect look. By using my folded hands and knuckles to help me raise myself from sitting and lying positions. Naturally, the knuckles' skin have toughened during the constant, daily, up-lifting weight processes. I am thankful that I am able to raise myself. So, I think less about the tough hand look. I simply try to keep my hands, legs, and feet moisturized with lotions or other emollients.

I often wish that I could receive cosmetic surgeries on my arms and legs. There are times when I do feel self-conscientious because of the many, many unsightly noticeable scars. Most of the scars are caused from falls. Some of them have appeared from trying to anchor my body from falling, thereby catching whatever piece of furniture to align myself. I have used many expensive across the counter scar/skin removers to no avail. My good rationale is that, no matter how my skin appears, I am moving around.

E. C. McCOLLUM-FLANIGAN

A. ACHES...PAINS...NERVE DAMAGES...MUSCLE TIGHTNESSES

About three years after the MS diagnosis, I began to have pain underneath my right shoulder blade. With x-rays and physical detailed therapy, the intermittent pain presently still occurs. I have experienced that when I readjust my back posture, by shifting my sitting and lying positions, within a short period of time, the pain is often lessened.

I also began to have excruciating left buttock pain. That very frequent pain often brought me to tears. The buttock pain did not go away completely with body shifting. Ironically, both pains began relatively near the same time. I saw my physician and described the pains. My physician examined me and prescribed some pain pills and showed me how to do some moderate stretching exercises as best as I could do them. Presently, while writing, sitting in a straight, somewhat ladder-backed chair, I am experiencing pain in three places. Below my right shoulder blade, my left buttock, and my right leg from the calf downward to my right foot, mingled with the tightness. My beloved husband purchased me some expensive rubbing ointment. The ointment helped from time to time.

I alternately used the special pain relieving ointment and the pills, trying to see which one worked.

I guess, both helped minimally. The pain pill prescription nor the ointment relieved the pain sufficiently as I had thought they would. The pills did contain a little codeine, too. The lack of effectiveness had to do with my immune system's intolerance to the MS enemy. So, I visited my physician again for the follow-up report. I was prescribed another prescription. With that prescription, I took two or three of the pills per day. Proudly to say, after about two or three days, the buttock pain went away off and on. Presently, I still suffer with the buttock pain and back pains sporadically. The pains are no jokes. Again, by shifting my position and taking my medication, the pain ceases more often that not.

What another irritating discomforting mess I was in. It was/is hard trying to get in a comfortable position to sleep, relax, or even sit. Lying on my left side, my buttock hurts. Lying on my right side, my back hurts. Lying on my stomach was not even comfortable. It was/is rough, because I do not fall asleep easily any way. Therefore, the best I could /can do is to lie on my back. I tried sleeping on a superior top of the line, orthopedic mattress, that my husband and I had purchased. I tried sleeping on a waterbed in another bedroom. Still seeking a good sleeping position, I tried sleeping on a king-sized cushioned couch, still searching for a comfortable position. Well, I can say that today by choice, I am still alternating among the three sleeping choices in my home. Redundantly, the common and sensible questions are; Why continue seeing physicians and taking medications to no avail? Why continue the periodic physical therapies to no avail, etc. because I know that I must follow recommendations for my own benefit, and I do fine.

Coincidently, another thing occurred near that time. Approximately three years after the MS' enemy's diagnosis, my dear husband had suffered critical pain and agitation in his right shoulder. Well, following his physician's recommendations of prescribed medications, physical therapy, an X-ray, an MRI, the true problem was spotted. My husband's rotator cuff was severely damaged (years of wear and tear of a professional truck driver, other freight system related work, and constant movements of right arms of hobbies, etc) Under going the only cure, my husband had rotator cuff surgery on his right shoulder. WOW! What a couple we made. My back, buttock, and sometimes the right side of my leg had discomforts. His right shoulder, arm, and hand also had discomforts. He had a very difficult time too, locating a good resting position throughout his long before and after surgery recuperating period. Who had to be whose caregiver? With GOD'S goodness and mercies, we helped each other and made out just fine. We shared our individual strengths and weaknesses.

B. DENTAL

Prior and since the MS diagnosis, I had/have observed and kept very good dental hygiene I have had a lot of expensive (insurance and out of pocket monies) dental work done that I do not remember all and every procedure that has been done for improvement of some dental upkeep.

Again, and ironically, how did I regularly take care of my teeth and still had lots of dental repairs? That is ironic and true! Why and how, again would be the questions.

From years of periodic extensive hygiene of cleanings, fillings, extractions, root canals, replacement bonding, and partials, have kept me occasionally busy in a dental chair. Within in the past two years, I have decided to stop getting filling repairs and root canals. Presently, anything that has to be repaired, I am getting extractions through oral surgery, and eventually up-dated partials.

Why? Remember my age. A few of my fillings are probably at least years old and will need to be repaired at some point. Therefore, I am at the point where I will simply get oral surgery and stop repeating the repairs of fillings and root canals. It is a real task getting my dentist, and probably any excellent dentist, to agree with this extraction method of good dental maintenance. Coincidentally also, somebody's research and statistics, recommends that MS patients should get metal fillings removed as soon as possible.

Basically, I think that dentists prefer patients to keep their natural teeth as long as possible. Plus, as long as there are repairs, there is more money for them. That really makes sense too, especially to professionals.

I am missing approximately eight or ten of my natural permanent teeth, since the age of six or something like that. No, no, no, I do not look like a snaggled-toothed clown. I am often told that I have a beautiful smile. Remember I have bonded teeth and a small partial replacement. They accommodate for my natural rear teeth that are missing. To my knowledge, the only thing that I failed to get was braces. Of course, braces were not popular in my circle during my younger years. You might know why as well as I do. But, do you know what? My husband and I financially paid our dues with braces for our sons during their proper times for teeth alignments too.

C. VISION

Very gratefully, I am working against the MS enemy's trying to attack my optic nerves. I do not and will not allow the intruder to cause me to have blurred vision or double vision. My eyes do not make small jerky movements. I definitely am able see in colors also.

About two years after the MS diagnosis, I developed a terrible eye allergy.

No, I do not think the enemy had control. Never had I suffered from any allergy disorder. One day I woke up with a very red, itchy, extremely puss filled right eye lid. I did the home eye wash remedy. Unfortunately, the eye had itched so much that I knew that I needed professional help. From my mirror feed back reflection, I wore a perfect natural Halloween disguise. My cornea was extremely red and surrounded by a black circle. It looked like I had been punched by a boxer.

The ophthalmologist examined, diagnosed, and explained to me what had happened.

Geographically, I reside in an area that is exceptionally high in pollution. I think the pollution count fluctuates in the purple, red, and orange zones very often. The main reason is because of the high and busy traffic in the component cites in the humungous metropolitan areas. This factor effects my specific area due to the constant wind shifts from the big metro area's traffic and factories residue, directly and heavily to my locale. YUK!

Along with the pollution damage, I had scratched the chronic itching, scarring my right cornea. What a real mess I caused too. After applying the prescribed antibiotic drops, and drops to help clear the redness, the eye felt and looked normal. However, because the blood vessels underneath the lid had been bruised, even today, looking in a bright make-up mirror, there is still a slight black-eye resemblance.

I am far-sighted, and that is good to me. Also, at my age, presbyopia has set in naturally. I wear reading glasses to read fine print. I wore prescribed reading glasses for years. Today, I simply wear over the counter reading glasses. They work just fine. So fine, that I have a pair in almost every room in my home, in my purse, and in my automobile, for my convenience. I also wear sun glasses to protect against bright light and the sun's glare on sunny days.

Medically, I also have prescription reading glasses, that I am wearing more and more of the time when reading. I really want to repress the enemy's attack on my optic nerves.

D. INSOMNIA

Insomnia has become a household word with me. It is aggravating because I know that natural sleep is a natural healer. Since retirement, I have all of the time in the world to take daily naps. Surprise! It does not happen to me that way. It is the sneaky intruder's fault. Occasionally, and very occasionally, I must say, that I may blink off no more than five to fifteen minutes. Upon awakening, I surprise myself that I did take a cat-nap.

I discussed my insomnia with my physicians. They explained that insomnia was/is a true side-effect of MS. The MS enemy loves this "no sleep game." It means that one has more conscience time to physically and mentally deal with misery. The physicians also stated that since I had retired, I now have some physically inactive periods during the day, as compared to the active use of my time while working and participating in some physical activities. Therefore, my body is really already rested daily, which may lead to less sleep needed.

My neurologist does prescribe enough sleeping medications to help eliminate the nightly insomnia. Now, the medication does work on the occasions that I take it. My problem is, I choose only to take it very seldom. Why? I do not want to become addicted to the medication nightly. What is wrong with my thinking when I complain that I wish that I was/am able to sleep nightly, so that I would have less time to feel miserable? I have the medication which allows me to fall asleep relatively quickly, and relatively longer hours. Yet, I refuse to take it nightly. I know, does that make a lot of sense? My warning to anyone who takes sleeping medication is, be sure to be in bed quickly after or before taking the medication. I have had a few bad experiences by taking the sleep medication and failed to immediately lie down. I do not remember what happened. The following mornings, upon awaking, I realized that I was in bed, but I was in my clothes from the previous days.

Luckily, for some strange reason, my younger son had been visiting. Therefore, he was available to help my husband physically get me upstairs to our bedroom. One occasion my grandchildren were also visiting and helped with the process of tucking me in.

That can be a weird and scary feeling. There was no excuse for my not going to bed, being knowledgeable of the could be severe and damaging consequences. There is one thing that I am super about. I never take the sleeping medication when I am home alone. No matter how bad I feel., I also tell my husband in advance the nights that I take the medication.

Of course, I shared this with my neurologist. He stated to me that when I did/do not desire to take a possibly addicted nightly sleeping pill, I could purchase an across the counter antihistamine which includes diphedryl, a mild sleeping ingredient. I now take two of those pills regularly. They work well too, and serve the purpose.

Occasionally, I will take a couple of tablespoons of over the counter extra strength P.M. cough syrup. Occasionally, I will drink a cup of specifically designated 'nerve, soothing, sleepy, caffeine free', hot tea before retiring for the night.

No, no, no, I do not try but one method at a time. I am very conscientious about not mixing medicines. I definitely read labels and warnings about negative drug interactions and side effects.

Again, why do I allow insomnia to rob me of nightly sleep when I have and know of various safe means of overcoming insomnia? I am very conscientious of trying not to load my system with unneeded substances. Even after taking a form of sleeping medicine, occasionally, I still do not fall immediately asleep. I have had a rare experience of becoming wide awake after taking the medication.

Presently, I can not remember what I had been doing or the variables that lead to the awake longer stages. Sometimes I have/do toss and turn for a while before going to sleep. Occasionally, I mentally count until all of the sheep have fallen asleep.

I am also very conscience of my next day's activities before I take a prescribed sleeping pill at night. This is because of one of the main warnings. The side effect warning reminds one to allow enough follow up sleeping time after taking the medication, not be overactive for a short safety period. A side effect of awakening too early is, one may be clumsy, inattentive, and sleepy.

Now, really, do I need any help at all in the clumsy department? I guarantee you, I do not need additional help in the clumsy department. I have passed the "Clumsiness 101" Class with an A+ average. I am still an active participant in the Class too. After taking the sleeping medication, I do feel very relaxed. Unfortunately, even taking the small milligram of sleeping medication, I will still only sleep, at the maximum, five or six hours. I do not double the recommended dose, no matter what. Those hours are not sound continuous sleep because the MS enemy makes sure that almost once nightly, I will have to have an urgent urine disturbance. But, do you know what? I would love to sleep straight through out the night, but, I am very thankful and grateful that the GOOD LORD allows me to wake up and use the bathroom properly, rather than wet my clothes, my linen, and possibly some part of my husband.

Most of the times, after rising to use my bedroom bathroom, I do return to bed and quickly fall asleep again, GOD is good. I am thankful also that I very rarely remember my dreams. When I do, they are quite small, unrecognizable, unrelated, minute nightmares. The nightmares do not bother me, because they are very rare and very short. So, I do not try to recall them and unscramble the unknown puzzles.

I have experienced a few times when I almost did not wake up from the bladder urgency in time to completely get to the bathroom without some uncontrolled drips. Luckily, my distance is short.

Incidentally, after my dismissal from the catastrophic CNS Hospital, and the removal of the attached catheter, I did use bed pads for a short personal experimental period, just to make sure that I would not damage my mattress. I had several bed pads left over from my in-patient stay.

Okay, I will try to keep the reading flowing on one subject. "Urine" is the next section.

I reiterate, sleep is a natural healer, and lends a temporary cover up to one's humanistic miseries.

I will always continue to praise and thank GOD, that I am okay and blessed!

E. INCONTINENCE/BLADDER DYSFUNCTION

Involuntary loss of urine causes real problems of bladder dysfunction to an individual. It is usually okay when an individual is hospitalized and temporarily wears a foley catheter or a diaper. A foley catheter is an indwelling catheter which stays in the bladder and drains urine at all times. It has a balloon on the end which holds it inside the bladder.

Quite often, with MS persons, it becomes part of a permanent "Bladder Program". This is a life style adaptation. It is never a life style change that one can push under the rug and say that it will get better in a little while. Luckily, there are pharmaceutical aids to help the big time problem.

Among the several kinds of incontinences, I was diagnosed with the "urge urinary incontinence", which involves the involuntary loss of urine associated with a very strong urge to urinate.

Before the enemy's intrusion, I had been a person who could retain my urine for hours after receiving a brain signal for release. "I gotta pee", meant to me that at some later time, eventually I would get around and take time out to use a restroom. During those unhealthy waiting and holding periods, the thought never occurred to me that I would have accidents, and I never did have accidents.

During those long time periods, back in the dark ages of my life, for many years, in an average day I would have drunk many cups of coffee and maybe a soda. My final cup of coffee would be a nightcap cup in bed. I had no thought at all that the coffee would keep me awake, and it did not keep me awake. It was like a sedative. With hind sight now, I would drink my nightly cup of black coffee propped upon a pillow, smoke a cigarette, make sure that the butt was exhausted, and fall right to sleep. I slept soundly throughout the night, unless some noise occurred loudly from a by-passing vehicle.

or some home activity caused me to be awake. The urge to use the bathroom during the night did not exist.

Okay, I am back on track with the subject. The following embarrassing urine accidents must be shared for a real true picture of urge urinary incontinence. When I got to go, I have got to go. I mean that I really have to go right then. The urge does not allow lollygagging around for any minute thing. There is absolutely no time for waiting around doing something else. No matter what I am doing, or no matter where I am, urine release is on its way when I receive my brain's message. More times than I would like to remember, like other sufferers of MS, the hurry is on.

Some super embarrassing times were in private, and unfortunately for me, some embarrassing times could have been in public. There is a feeling that one has to be there to know the personal turmoil that is suffered when urine is about to involuntarily escape. I am sure that the horrible MS devil has a notorious field day. Later, I will share the way that I conquered the monster, most of the times, and brought the MS enemy down from its maximum strategy moves.

Remember, I had spent two or three years with difficult and very strange, nearly unexplainable discomforts happening to me physically before I got a diagnosis. Therefore, body functions had begun to dysfunction causing me to wonder and do personal research seeking some facts and causes of what was happening to my once healthy body.

My hind-sight memory, as menopause was setting in, before the MS diagnosis, during the period that I was constantly taking boucoup medical tests, I had experienced enough bladder/bowel discomforts to modify the liquids that I consumed. The very first incident that I remember was while I was unlocking my home door to enter. Before I realized what was really happening, I sped fastly to my bathroom.

Normally, I would have taken my time and got to the bathroom in time. I had a very strange and uncomfortable feeling for that experience to be happening to me without my consent.

Another earlier time, the accident happened at work. I made it to the bathroom, but for some strange and unusual reason, I was unable to get my pants' zipper unzipped in time. I finally just yanked the stuck zipper down. Can you imagine walking out of the restroom with front and back pee damages showing on your clothing? I pray not, and very thankful I did not.

For some unknown reason, I never wore that pants suit again. It was pretty and relatively new. I know that was poor rationale. The accident almost happened to my body, not because of the suit. But, you know what, the lamed zipper did play a part of the delay. The new pants suit had to go. I did not need anything to remind me of that bad experience.

Contrary things happening like that can really work on one's mind and self morale. Now, what is going on? This cannot be happening to me. I was a person who had been in control of my organ functions.

Around that time and the embarrassing almost accidents began to happen often. I shared this with my gynecologist. He examined me and stated that he did not see anything wrong in spite of having done the routine bladder tacking/tucking after performing my hysterectomy successfully. He then referred me to a urologist, just to begin to nip my nagging bladder problem in the bud.

The urologist performed several cytologists tests. He told me that the kugel exercises probably would not be beneficial. He prescribed some bladder control pills and told me to return if I did not see a change in urine urges after taking the medication for a while.

The pills seemed to help somewhat, I also began monitoring my liquid intakes of caffeine in coffee, sodas, and plain water, especially when I had plans of not being at home.

I then covered my pride and purchased as recommended, a pack of urine bladder pads. I had seen the idea advertised on television. I had noticed pamphlets about them in the urologist's office. If you have not been there, try to image how degrading and embarrassing it was for me to purchase the pads. I medically realized later, and bladder questions from my neurologist, that unbeknown to me, the sneaky, devil MS enemy was silently sliding in my body and intruding. A slight opportunity was there for the scoundrel, since I had had a bladder tacking and tucking and would definitely not notice it sliding in.

In initially purchasing my first urinary pads, first of all, it took some time for me to read and compare several name brands to try to decipher what was being offered. I was looking for the pads that would consume the most wetness.

During my reading info, a familiar shopper was by passing and stopped to chit-chat briefly. I noticed that she had glanced at what I was busy doing. I made a lame excuse and stated something like. "I really do not know what I am doing, since I am buying the pads for someone else." What a liar I had momentarily become to try to save face from embarrassment.

After making a blind choice, I covered the pack of pads in the cart with other items I was purchasing. Occasionally, I will presently do that. Why? Maybe it is a form of denial just in case some acquaintance should see me with them. I would honestly quickly explain the particular purchase if I would be alone with an acquaintance at those times, instead of having other shoppers listening. I really do not care, I am following medical directions.

Through experimenting with various pads, and almost being unable to make it to a restroom in the nick of time, I learned what pads work best for me. Yes, I still occasionally have to hurry when I get the bladder urge and cannot locate a restroom quickly. I have a mental comfort zone by locating restrooms first.

Yes, I have had the urges in the most dignified places. It has happened in my automobile; in a church while standing after sitting for a while; in grocery and department stores while hurriedly walking to the far away restroom; walking in the streets; on a plane while waiting for someone to exit from the restroom; on a cruise ship at sea when I could not locate a restroom while exploring on the ship; a few times in my home; standing up or getting in my car; waiting in line in a public restroom while waiting for an available stall…Aren't those enough times for anyone to get a wake up call? It is unexplainable and horrible to know what is going to embarrassingly happen big time and not be able to make any corrections to avoid the situation that I always know is about to happen.

What do I do in those awful times? I keep walking to the restroom. I silently pray, "JESUS, please let me get to an available stall in the restroom." Most of the times I do make it to the restroom before the flood gates really let go, because most of the places I go, I have already gotten familiar with the restrooms' locations I have learned to wear black, navy, or camouflaging patterns of pants, whether long, short, capri, or any other style. Thankfully now my associates do not aggravate or make me feel bad when I always locate the closest restroom areas while visiting all places. No, my associates, whether family members or friends understand and help locate the restroom in first time places visited.

Thanks for reading my story. I do realize that it may sound downright uncaring and stupid at times of the loss of control of nerve messages misread from the brain and failing to receive proper relay and feedback. No, I am definitely not saying that my readers are unsure of the CNS. Of course not. But like me, there are many, many subjects that I am definitely unsure about. Trust me, it is no joke to live with interrupted messages going to and from the brain. Think about how frustrating it is when one's computer has a glitch and progress is slowed, confused, or even stopped. However, it is with the utmost gratitude to be manageably surviving.

Some common questions that I have been asked are:

1) Why wait or procrastinate going to the restroom upon the initial urge? I do not wait. As stated earlier, usually when the urge comes, it is already time for urine to pass.
2) Why consume so much liquid? I purposely do not consume lots of liquids, in spite of knowing that my body needs certain amounts of liquids to aid with my metabolism.

Later, in the next chapter, notice how the intake of liquids pose a real dilemma.

3) Why do I get caught up in a bladder dysfunction? I did/do not get caught up in it. That very disgusting unwanted intruder MS, got very rudely got caught up in me.

So, due to the CNS as well as the PNS, the disease of MS chooses, plays. and cares less, about the havoc it purposely causes to the nervous and muscular functions controlled systems. The enemy's goal is for every system to lose control.

Improving and winning against the MS enemy, require changes in my life style routines daily. I am still blessed because I am not cauterized or wearing adult diapers. I have learned to modify or downsize my wardrobe coloring. You know what? That is great because dark pants colors are basic and very common and always fashionable anyway and anywhere.

F. IRRITABLE BOWEL SYNDROME

Living with irritable bowel is a big problem within itself. During the approximate year and a half period while I was seeking a diagnosis for the unknown malady, and thus forth evermore, and occasionally in the present., I have some experiences to share. Please allow me to share a few horrendous experiences, that may read like something x-rated or from the twilight zone.

Obviously, a bowel problem is worse than a bladder problem. It is one that can not be disguised through camouflaging clothing and odors. How did my life get to this up-side- down predicament?

The notorious MS intruder caused me to loose a lot of nerve and muscle control of my colon. In other words, sometimes I am not able to one hundred percent control the normal colon/rectal feeling signifying the message from my brain that it is time to eliminate waste. Thus, I am able to feel when the time comes, but I am unable to wait and control the movements to stop passing for long periods.

Again, I hope that I am letting others knew that they are not alone bearing the MS monster's tricks.

I really had no idea that the final processes in my digestive tract, would become so malfunctioning to cause almost embarrassing problems. When I first experienced that I was definitely having problems, I took a few across the counter laxatives. I thought that the sluggishness was just a temporary something. The only time that I had had a bowel problem was when the former related fibroid tumors had pressed too forcefully against my bladder and colon. That malfunction had been somewhat corrected when I had the hysterectomy.

Once I shared this new bowel problem with an elderly relative, she told me to try drinking senna tea. The laxatives, and especially the senna tea worked. However, I had another big problem. I was unable to control when they would want to work.

I tried planning the timing when they would work, so that I would be in my home bathroom at the end of the day. I tried planning so that I would be in my home bathroom at the beginning of the day. Both plans failed more times than I would like to remember.

When I faced the fact that I had to get a handle on the "Bowel Program", I made an appointment with a gastroenterologist. I had several appointments with her and several tests. I had a colon test to check and see if there were developing polyps growing on any sections of my intestines. There were not any. There was another test where I was able to see the monitor of my lower digestive tract, as my gastroenterologist and her assistant inserted a small flexible instrument in my rectum to my stomach, trying to see if maybe there were minute blockages that were keeping my bowels from functioning normally. The results revealed that my intestines, (small or large, I do not remember) had some with noticeable curves, length maybe thereby, causing my bowels to pass in an irregular way. Add that irregularity to what the MS enemy was doing. Again, the enemy could very easily gain points in its game.

I was prescribed a clear like laxative that was powder and had to be mixed with a gallon of tap water. I had to drink one to three glasses of it daily. It worked, but not smoothly as I had thought it would. It also caused all kinds of bubbling and growling noises from my stomach.

Once I felt really neausially ill and shaky while monitoring students. Luckily, they were involved with a locker break, and did not notice me or I would have probably made the evening local news if I had really overtly been sick

Once my husband and I were out of town, in a popular cafeteria buffet line, and bingo! The only warning I received was a short bubbling growl, in the restroom recuperating so long that my husband sent a waitress in to check on me. That was really nice of him.

Embarrassingly, I was on my way out of the restroom when the waitress showed up. I thanked her and told her that I had felt ill. Truly, I had felt some minutes of emotional distress, and physically, I could not regroup, rapidly from what felt like neaseau and possibly the beginning of some diarrhea synmotaneously about to happen.

Regardless of how frequently my bladder and bowel get my immediate attention, there is nothing, doing those occurrences, easy to emotionally accept. Sure I am a veteran now. Although I try very hard to plan ahead, so my functions timings will be on task, and hopefully, I will be in a right place, at the right times. I am currently on a self-evaluation of possibly an "8 from 1(low) to 10(high)", with my Bowel Program medication, and conquering the enemy.

I make absolutely sure that I use the bathroom each time before leaving home, a store, a restaurant, a church, from visiting someone else's home, and nearly all outings.

I use that precaution just in case I get caught in bumper to bumper traffic jams, or some other time consuming places. Most of the time my precaution works. Still, remember, when, "I gotta go, I have gotta go", regardless of the circumstances. Are there any witnesses to this speedy, hurry up experience? Now, you know that you are not alone.

Welcome to the club! I am always thankful to GOD for answering my prayers of allowing me the privilege of being in the right place at the right time, instead of being embarrassed somewhere else. Sometimes I am so grateful that I have shed a few tears of gratitude. What? Why? I can remember where I have come from. I know how degrading and embarrassing circumstances might happen. "Been there, done that," unfortunately many times. I thank my readers for bearing with me through this very life sustaining experience.

Okay, what is the big deal about a natural body function? Please do not allow the MS instigator to try to fool you. That inhuman MS character can try to make disaster in one's life.

One of the most different aspects of the beginning of the irritable MS bowel syndrome, was accepting the reality.

For a short while I blamed the irrital bowel syndrome from all of the common shared opinions, it seemed like, almost everybody, who was somebody, had had a hysterectomy. I knew young and older

MULTIPLE SCLEROSIS, THE HORRENDOUS, NOTORIOUS, UNINVITED, INTRUDER

women who had had the surgery, and still presently do, before I had the surgery.

I questioned this with my gynecologist, my gastroenterologist, and my neurologist.

They assured me that, a few days a week is an average normal bowel movement for some people. No, there may not be a "carved in stone" for everyone.

There are some people who regularly defecate once a week. Wow! Can you believe that? Once a week after consuming seven days of solids and liquids, at least three times a day, and digesting junk food too. WHOA! Obviously there are different strucks for different folks.

Although, the obnoxious MS intruder, has caused me to lose a lot of sensitiveness, I do have rectal signals. I just can not always predict the quick or sluggish signals. Like with incontinence, when I receive the stimuli prompting, there is absolutely no time for waiting around.

Try to image what happens when I get to a restroom and there is not an available stall. I would not want those insecurities to happen to my worst enemy.

I think that those are attacks or some types of MS exasperations. My physicians had asked me about the latest attacks I had experienced. I did not know what an attack meant then.

I definitely know now, in several areas of dysfunctions.

I will share a few other events when the MS enemy had me at times of disadvantages for me. Once, I had a scary attack at work. While I was standing and doing a science demonstration/lecture, suddenly and very excruciatingly, a sharp pain traveled from my rectum down to the side of my right leg, to my right foot. Oh, what a predicament. Again, I would have made the nightly news, big time if I had had an accident. I stood as still as I could stand. Added to my already off balanced stance, it was not easy. The pain came in quick intervals, somewhat like mini child labor contractions. Luckily, I was near my classroom door. I quickly told a dependable and reliable student to go to the board and write the names of anyone who was disorderly. I did not even have time to alert the teacher next door, to keep an eye on my class. I was out of the room in a flash. My immediate thought was to get to the first restroom around the corner. I was also very aware, and very conscientious of leaving my students unattended. That was not something I would do, not by law, and not by my own responsibility to them. I did not have time to coordinate that fast necessary emergency move.

Thankfully, I barely made it before disaster happened. I would have really been on the headline evening news with that performance.

I felt piercing, excruciating pain traveled from my rectum down my right leg to my right foot.

Another time, as I was rising from my couch, I realized that I was unable to walk the very short distance to my steps. So, I got on the floor and scooted from the couch to the stairs. I painstakingly crawled the steps. When I finally crawled to the bathroom, I was unable to lift myself from the floor to the stool's ream. I tried again. Both times, the lack of being unable to heist myself from the floor to the stool scared me.

The inability to walk brought a very serious flash back to me.

After much scuffling and up-lifting trials, using my arms and fists trying to raise myself to the stool, I was unsuccessful. Finally, after doing many trials, I caught the edge of the face bowl cabinet and with all of the strength I could muster, I lifted enough to sit on the stool.

I was afraid to get in the shower in lieu of falling. Therefore, I took a good sponge bath by sitting on the adjacent stool. My husband was then home. With his help, I got to my bed. I had trouble, but with his assistance, I got there.

I had bed pads left from my previous hospital stay. I lay and slept on one of them for security. I had the feeling that maybe I would not be able to get to the bathroom if needed. I did some serious praying. Thank you, LORD! I was able to walk and the pain was gone the next morning!

Following the next episode of my saga, I went to my gastroenterologist. I felt tinges of intermittent rectum aches and twitches. I was referred to a metro hospital for another specific colon-something exam. Why I have forgotten the name, I do not know. I think it was a colonoscopy. As an out put-patient, I was given an enema. I used the bathroom, afterward the test was given. I lay on my left side. Two staff members assisted each other. Some thing was inserted and there was more monitor recording.

For medication prior to receiving the test, my gastroenterologist told me to buy a cheap enema, then drain the medication out, and fill the bottle with tap water. Later, after the good test result, whatever the test was for, now I have forgotten, and I did not check the record of the specific test taken. She prescribed the pre-stated water/powder medication to help with bowel regulation.

I have had to learn how to live through this dramatic and traumatic body and life style change through lots of prayer, through lots of people support, and through lots of trials and errors. The Bowel Program is another major function that can not be shoved under the rug in denial. Being faced with difficulties that have to be accepted, and positively coordinated for livelihood, is a must, without absolutely and positively no doubt and few procrastinations.

Life makes and takes some mountainous bumps and perilous twists. Becoming and enduring adaptations, modifications, and adjustments to one's life styles changes are factors for success. Some strategies are rough and the goings do get tough. It is all about doing what it takes to remain mobile and independent as possible. It is about showing the MS intruder that no weapon formed against me is going to prosper. It will learn that its weapons will not work without failures, for me.

"GOD is good all the time, and all the time GOD is good!"

PSALM 4: 1
Hear me when I call, O GOD of my righteousness, THOU hast enlarged me when I was in distress; have mercy upon me and hear my prayer.

G. ALTERNATIVE...HOLISTIC...PROGRAMS

The dynamic and innovative medical board certified professionals try to do everything possible to enhance patients to acquire wellness.

The list can go on and on to unlimited recommendations, trials and errors of what one should do to improve medical deficiencies. Often, all approved medications and therapies have been applied and a patient may still remain at square one.

Generally, when this happens, or in another cliché interpretation, "When the doctor shakes his head and slowly walks away", a suffering patient or members of the patient's family will search other ways to try to help the sick one. Many alternative medicines or medical alternates are on the market on every corner, or in any magazine advertisements, the testimonies of how such and such, and this and that have helped almost any area of common sicknesses.

To me, and foremost, my healing has to come from JESUS CHRIST, my LORD and SAVIOR. I believe that GOD uses medical professionals as His instruments to stand in the gaps for HIS healing works. HE gives them the intelligence to study, practice, and perform miraculous advancements and successes through HIS guidance, goodness, and mercies. Notably, those advances are not solely limited to the medical field. There are broadened and perfected remedies in every field.

Today, I may not remember every alternative method I have tried. I may not remember every alternative lecture or seminar that I have attended. There were many. The main objectives were to find something legally, that could make me feel better. No matter what methods I tried, no matter how expensive they were, I never, ever forgot to ask, praise and thank my Almighty for HIS healing. I do that everyday. I ask GOD to replace every diseased cell in my body with healthy, normal, functional cells. I pray for HIS gift of patience in waiting for my healing to come to me.

For insomnia, I was told by a physical therapist that I could use the aromatic natural fragrance of lavender. I could lightly spray it near my pillow or in my bedroom. I could purchase an aromatic lavender fragrance candle to burn for a short time in my bedroom. The main point was/is that it has to be 100% natural or a derivative of a 100% natural herb. I did purchase the natural spray fragrance. When I think about it, I sometimes spray it near my side of the bed and lightly on the underside of my pillow.

Does it work? I do not really know because it is time for me to fall asleep anyway. Okay, I did say earlier that it was hard for me to naturally fall asleep, it usually is, so per change the lavender aroma does help.

Also for peace, restlessness/insomnia tranquility, irritable bowels, and other irritations, I have often drunk specific nerve soothing caffeine-free herbal teas. Some examples were; chamomile, sleepy time, hops, valerian, peppermint, mint. ginger, senna leaf, cranberry, and on and on.

I have tried various herbal rubs and salves to try toning down the tightness and heat in my legs and feet. Those rubs included; spiritually anointed olive oil, natural emu derived oils, oils with blue herbal ingredients, mineral oil based substances, oils with coco butter and aloe vera, and many others. I have somewhat, usually on short time periods, modified my diet. I tried eating healing foods with more grains and fiber contents. I tried eating more fruits and green vegetables. I briefly tried omitting red meats. However, that went over like a lead balloon because often I simply want to eat sirloin in steaks or roasts. I tried wheat breads and crackers. But, since adulthood, I have always preferred wheat grains over white grains anyway.

I tried alternate pills recommended by naturalists. I tried drinking specially prepared juices containing bran, aloe vera, and other natural ground fibers. I tried drinking at least eight glasses of water daily to help regulate my bowels, my metabolism, and enhance my skin. Drinking that much water, along with prune, apple, or orange juices was not the problem. The problem was the increased urine flow and bladder dysfunctions. I mentioned this to a nurse and her reply to me was that by consuming that much liquid daily could cause my kidneys to become over-activated. That made sense to me. Now, I had acquired another controversial dilemma. In order to help naturally regulate irritable bladder and bowel syndromes, I must drink enough liquids that would over act other organs.

I have tried many things, but when I have not seen or felt improvements in at least three to four months, I discontinue what I had begun. Yes, I definitely always continue taking my prescription medications. I know, since I am trying alternatives and taking prescriptions, how do I really know which method is working or not working? I do not know. I do know that I have taken my prescriptions consistently and longer. So, I can assume that if and when I take alternatives and began to feel noticeable difference, then the alternative method may be working. That has not happened. I am very reluctant and I do not plan on discontinuing my prescribed medications until my miracle healing appears.

I remember hearing on the media and reading in the paper about a very few MS patients who daily smoke a joint of marijuana, and drink a shot of alcohol, and feel wonderful, or just lying to say that they will live happily ever after. No, and definitely no, that method is not for me. I will not try that method no matter what. Sure, I grew up during the Hippy Era, but I did not indulge, and I will not indulge now to help the MS menace cause other problems for me. That is simply and factually, not the way for me to go. I can only visualize adding further chronic insult, severe damage, and chaos to the already resulting injury that way.

I try to walk as often and as much as I am able to do so. I ride my stationery bike and walk on my treadmill not as much or as long as I should. I was taking aquatic exercises at least twice a week for awhile. But, presently, I am on a lazy hiatus from that, due to another foot tripping injury.

I tried reflexology. My feet were dipped in melted, as hot as I could take it, paraffin. Then the therapist put some thin plastic disposable socks on my feet. About fifteen minutes later, the paraffin was removed. Next was the reflexology and electric acupuncture treatments They did not cure anything, but, wow! it was so relaxing just to receive the soothing massage reflexology treatments. I would experience that soothing invigorating type of treatment forever, if I could do so. I plan to continue that particular treatment periodically because it is extremely soothing. I do not have to do any thing but relax and receive the automatic massage heat treatment lying on my back.

I try to use an alternative method in thinking cognitively positive. Sometimes my roller coaster emotional sensitivities get in the way. However, I can ignore the MS enemy trying to pull me mentally down, and I pray for control. That works. It usually cost me a few crocodile tears and mental bashing, but I know that GOD'S mercy is on the way. After, a short time, usually unconsciously, I will realize that that frustration has passed.

I have learned and I am still learning to use alternative ways of performing and completing personal tasks. I know, that's not a holistic coverage. However, for my personal progress, I can put other little tasks under the same umbrella of alternative coverage.

1st JOHN 5:14 & 15

14) And this is the confidence that we have in HIM, that, if we ask, any thing according to HIS will, HE heareth us;15) And if we know that HE heareth us, whatsoever we ask, we know that we have the petitions that we desire of HIM.

E. C. McCOLLUM-FLANIGAN

X. EMOTIONAL ROLLER COASTER

FEAR//MINOR DEPRESSION-GUILT-HAPPINESS-
SADNESS—SHAME—
COGNITIVE EFFECTS—REALITY, ETC.

PSALM 143:8
The LORD is gracious and compassionate, slow to anger and rich in love.

PSALM 147: 3
He heals the brokenhearted and binds up their wounds.

You are invited to ride along with me on my wishy-washy typical roller coaster exhilarant adventure. I do try to spend most of my time, on the height, soaring, rather than shuttering in the depth. Either place can become a very repetitive, and bumpy ride. I can not say that the ride is free. There is no down payment, but it sometimes costs me plenty. It can even have weekly installments consequences. It may not be too understandable for me to say, but the roller coaster ride is a main side effect of the MS's enemy's tricks and temporary spastic afflictions. Sometimes the ride is with tears, sometimes with cheers, and even sometimes with fears.

To get to the core of my saga of sad emotions, would be a single best seller in itself alone. Since, this is about how the dreadful, notorious, horrendous, MS, snuck in and changed my lifestyle, the ride is often very treacherous. So please get on board, because the MS enemy is a very devious, co-rider, silent pest. No, it was and forever will be a looser with me. But, some changes had to be made because of the pest.

Ordinarily, like in other people lives, some emotional issues and dramas overlap in my life, with or without the MS intruder. Realistically, changes in emotions are humanistic characteristics of life. Before the official MS diagnosis, again, hindsight let me know that the intruder was beginning to acclimate in its stolen dwelling. I felt some noticeable physical ailments that I could not explain or be knowingly justify. My associates knew that I was not my usual one-hundred percent well-rounded self.

There was not a drastic or real noticeable one day change. Changes began to accumulate and repetitive, that showed me the red flag. I just know that my physical and emotional demeanor slightly fluctuated. No, I did not deprive my students of their education, On contraire, I think that I became a more dedicated, if that was possible, (smile) educator. Some of my family and many of my close associates, including students, observations, knew what I had told them up-front about my physical state.

I appreciated everyone's concerns. I was asked, "What did the doctor say"? so often and so much, that that inquiry became a little frustrating. At times I had some incompetent feedback expressions. I did not feel good about my unanswered comments and inquiries to them. After so much negative comments concerning the physicians not being able to tell me what was wrong with me, I really did not know how to relay a good logical or rational reply to my associates, or to me.

I just listened to comments and suggestions about what I could have, should have, and would have done. Because, I heard those things so often, I did get a little down often, about not knowing what was wrong with me. Although people cared about me, and I truly cared/care that they do care, but I was tired of their inquisitive third degrees when I could not answer. Everyone was very nice and supportive to me.

As stated previously, I know, I too would think, "Why is this author saying it again, when he/she knows that the information has been stated." Well, it is about properly fitting the pieces to the puzzle congruently. Now, the day that I had gotten off work early to receive the lumbar puncture, I was mentally over-ready to get a definite diagnosis. I was not expecting to be informed that I had a terminal illness. I thought that when I would receive a diagnosis for the malady, a cure for whatever was wrong, would be on the way very soon. I thought that with specific and proper medications, oral, or some type of possible cortisone injections, plus maybe some physical therapy, I would return to my normal self. I had done a lot of personal research associated with my experienced ailments. I failed to program my mind that maybe I had an incurable something. Not, multiple sclerosis, I was a healthy conscientious person. I somewhat understood the complexity of the brain, spinal cord, the CNS and the PNS.

I had taught Life Science in middle school for years. My short coming was the denial that I would have some illness of MS magnitude.

I was not rude to people's inquisitiveness. I too, am inquisitive, and I too, know that I would have asked and asked someone about his or her status and demeanor. I heard, not through gossip, but in hearing proximity of others conversations, or specifically told to me that I should straighten up and walk like I normally use to do. I heard that I should hold my urine for a little while, instead of trying to seek attention by going to the bathroom when everyone had settled for any given program. I heard that no one was going to feel sorry for me on my self imposed pity pot. I heard that I should eat this or that and start a daily exercise routine. I was told that I was hypocritically judgmental by expressing my opposite opinions, when I disagreed with some others opinions.

I think that I know what a reader may suspect right about now. Maybe this author is a cantankerous, hypocritical, self-righteous attentions seeking wreck. No, I think absolutely not. I am pretty much a low-key, realistic, compassionate, unselfish, and giving individual. Constant positive oral feedbacks, from all kinds of acquaintances, in all kinds of situations, have let me know that I am not such a bad person with a hateful demeanor. No, I am also not a pompous jack.

I have heard that maybe I just wanted to sit at home. No, I did not. I enjoyed what I did. Was I going to be a burden to the family? No, I am not. In spite of being told that maybe I should be very grateful that somebody took away from their personal time to take care of me I really want to know how often and when did that happen. How long was I going to pretend that I felt bad? Never, because I never pretended illness anyway. Yes, I am off my rocker, if I feel that people who made those comments are supportive and loving acquaintances. No, I did/do not ever think that I would have to watch my back against them and the enemy too. Those are not compassionate statements, but they are very true statements to me.

I do face the fact that sometimes the people that one may need the most, will often not show up or call, just to say. "How are you doing, or do you need something?" I am guilty of that negligence too. For there are a few sick or shut-in persons in my church and community that I have failed to communicate or visit in a long while. Thus, I am guilty of that "no contact" to them also.

What seems like a lack of concern can really emotionally hurt. On the other side, too much concerned like constant interference would cause me some stress too. Okay, what do I really want from people? I know that my family and friends are here for me. However, I am so thankful that I am able to do almost anything that I need to be done. But, I have had pity-pot down sides of the roller coaster and asked myself, "Does any body really care and want to know how I really feel about the plight that this MS mess causes? Can't I just respectfully disagree to agree with some others opinions without being vocally bashed? Do I always have to bear someone else's short comings? Do I always have to be the person that makes mistakes? It is so easy for me to become sensitive and cry an awful lot. Now that is the MS monster's fault. Crying is not an abrupt response that I did before the MS enemy's attack. I was told that no one wanted to talk with me because all I would do is cry like a baby. Big deal, I hope that I do not treat people that way.

I was asked why didn't I wear this or that type of shoes in aid me in walking better? Why didn't I wear support hoses? Why didn't I simply use a wheelchair all of the time, since I said that my feet and legs were miserable.

To the knowledge of my research, MS/is was not inherited, and I had not known of any one on my paternal nor my maternal sides of the family with any illness similar to the MS mess. What horrible sins had I committed to be reaping what I had sown? Were those statements and questions voiced from my family, friends, or my foes? I forgive them, and pray that they forgive me for being my inquisitive self. I know that they are caring. Unfortunately, I do not always forget, like I should. I know that I should not allow myself to get on the lower end of my roller coaster. Gratefully, I definitely allow myself to get back up again.

One truthful reason that I have a hard time forgetting is because, when I am on a very smooth ride, and I move on out of the things that are emotional and very hurting challenges to me, something or someone always do or say something that reactivates my emotional pains. Every once in a while, it has appeared like the reversions were spoken on purpose. I think that that is simply the way life is for anyone. My thoughts were/are that I really did/do know a lot of retaliative people, when they were/are unable to deal with their own short comings. Then, they must put the monkey on someone else's back for personal rationales. Some minute things just happened on one of my real MS low days. Hearing incidents shared in my MS Group, lets me know that I am not alone with crying emotions. Once again, those are just normal human thoughts.

I do not mind having, counseling or psychological help. To me, almost anyone will have some type of analyst and counseling for something. I love them, and I know that they love me also. I definitely know that one can not speak candidly to people who misinterprets conversations and visually retaliate to cover and boost up their shortcomings and insecurities. Okay, this is a bunch of contradictory stuff. Either I have love and support or I do not. My emotions play havoc with it too.

E. C. McCOLLUM-FLANIGAN

There are some true merits to some comments, assumptions, and accusations in life with the enemy. That seems to be what life is. Sometimes I tend to carry unneeded and obsolete extra baggage from constant flashback reminders. I admit, that is my fault. I must forgive and forget.

What do I mean? I mean some statements that had caused me critical emotional hurt, will be similar and interpreted by me to be in on uncaring way. Why? Sometime I gave a lot of punch lines in response to negative behaviors and actions that I do not agree with. I feel that there are times when people must be able to agree to disagree. Not being able to do so can cause big problems sometimes. Every one has opinions.

I know that I am a giving person. Except for telling my husband, I like to remain anonymous in most of my monetary donations. I really enjoy giving to others, deeds, transportation at gas cost, parking fees, and money as often and as much as I can afford in order to help a few others when they are in financial immediate pinches. I share my donations from my heart, or I would not be so giving. Jokingly, I tell my family members that when they get back on their feet, with big time bucks, they had better remember me. No, I definitely do not hound them to repay me. Some times they repay a little. They know that I do not expect pay back. I know that they did not have any money when they needed it, any way, so why would I badger them. Not me.

My husband and I are always there for our sons and their families. We are still parents, even to adult children. Yes, they do have occupations and good careers, their own places to live, and financial obligations in the norm. They are good guys. One is married and the other is divorced. We have great times with our daughter-in-law, our ex-daughter-in-law, and our older grand son's mother.

I am accountable for my downfalls. Even when others tell me the negative ways that they think I behave, speak, and misinterpret others and get an attitude. But, I stand to be corrected. When something effects someone, is not that a personal something? Okay, if I know that, what is my problem? Even when I was/am experiencing a MS down side. What kind of ego boosting, self proclaimed, self-righteous denial mode do I like to remain in?

Once I was diagnosed with MS, then retired, and hospitalized, my husband was/is exceptionally supportive. In the past and, during the present, and in the future, I know that I can depend on him to help me through the horrible MS battle. It is always very comforting to live with that security.

We do lots of spiritual, fun, and compatible things together. We also attend lots of adventurous enlightening programs together. Often some of the Grandchildren are with us on our adventures. WOW! Coincidentally, traveling, riding around, have always been a part of our marriage style.

Those things were frequently occurring before our sons were born, also, with our sons, and presently without our adult sons. We continue to go on our "field trip," excursions and outings as much, and as often as we choose to do so. Sometimes the Grandchildren on our present adventures too. What great field trip excursions we experience with the Grandchildren!

I feel that best way to correct a mistake or error is to tell someone what he or she has done incorrectly. Accusations and any types of harassments, do not justify a wrong. The wrong issues have to be specifically voiced in a mature and suggestive correct manner. How else can the wrongs be righted?" One should get with the program unselfishly and successfully walk the wounded through corrections. When a person is told that he/she has erred, the person who tells he/she that, should be mature enough to share specific corrections ASAP. When not knowing questions happen to me, I want specific acknowledgements and suggestions to correct my short comings. I want them, at the time of offense. I do not want to have to ponderely unknowing make guesses.

Sometimes, my emotions may turn a little flip-flop, when I think that I may receive a little compliment and encouragement more than discouragement. I get compliments almost every where I go, all of the time from all ages and sexes. I tell them, "Thank you, and move on." Remember I never, ever desire or want to present myself as a pompous person. I also naturally return compliments to my family and everyone from time to time.

So, what is the big deal? Absolutely nothing. I just shared a wishy-washy thought. I think every individual has or will experience at least a few wishy-washy thoughts at some little particular time in his or her life. No, I do not think that I am judgmental by stating what others will experience in their lives. I choose to think that I am realistic.

The MS monster does have an effect on my sensitivity. It takes its toil. I would like to think that I do not allow the enemy to cause me so much physical and mental discomforts. But, since I feel discomforts, who is really calling the shots?

I have been in conversations, and I have been told that I need to be quiet and shut up. No one knows how that statement can get my attention. Truly, I know that those are just conversational lingoes. I know from my traumatic hospitalization period, and a person that I have met in my MS Group that some MS patients are unable to speak and do remain "shut up" permanently. That is why when I hear "shut up", it now has a new meaning to me.

I was/am saddened when I think that I am during helpful things and then I hear that the helpful tasks cause harm. I do know that my help, is really help, although the persons that I may be helping at those rare times, will choose to try to save their own face rather than show gratitude. It is then that I will receive a cut down more than I will receive gratitude. I have learned to live without hearing compliments, gratitude, or encouragement on those occasions. Why? I choose to think that they know. Now, you may think that this may happen to me because, of some attitude problem. Sure, a good question can be, "What have you ever done for others lately?

I have told my family that I never want to become a burden to others. I do not like the thought of the idea, but, realistically, I do not want to have to change caregivers and caretakers lives to accommodate my survival inabilities 24/7. I wish happiness and peace for them too. There are plenty assistant living institutions in my area. Hopefully, they would be affordable too. Yes, I still feel confident and proud to say that this MS idiotic enemy will not get me to that point. I believe in my JESUS. I really am grateful for their love, patience, help, care giving, and kindness as I need them.

I have been told that I have made some failures and wrong choices at times. What times? Who has not? I have no specific pros or cons from the sources of those accusations. I try to be up-lifting and compassionate to and for others, in spite of thinking that maybe I cause more harm to them than help. Do I believe that? No, I do not. Sometimes, I simply just allow myself to be a little bit of a scapegoat for others. I am around or mingling with too many associates who always compliment and tell me how great I am. I believe them. Why do my emotions shift gears then? My honest reply is, I do not always agree with others opinions, that appear negative to me. There are always two sides to everything. I thank GOD that HE sustains my mobility.

When I rarely think about some of the MS mess, maybe it is playing its game big time, thereby causing problems that I do not see. Maybe some of my limits do get in the way for others. In the way of what? I am not told. I can play an excellent game. I just do not know the game rules.

Following the MS diagnosis, it seemed like when I needed an emotional boost the most, both sons acquired some automobile grief and restrictions. Both? Yes, sadly to say, at different times, but both made some driving negative choices. Luckily, I was not dependent on them for transportation to get here and there. I felt their pain for their driving short comings. My husband and I helped both of them with expensive automobile driving tickets' financial disasters. I really needed to have adult give and take conversations with my sons. They did help me. However, they too were facing their on licenses driving temporary consequences. Both of them had paid for popular automobiles. What good is it to own an automobile when it is in some county's pound yard because of accumulated traffic offenses? Why? Simply by a few consecutively times of not observing driving laws. Trust me, they were taught and practiced safely, in the correct ways to honor the driving laws.

Presently, they are legally and more cautiously on the road again. Much gratitude goes to my daughter-in-law for chauffeuring her husband to and from work and around.

Were we able to console each others? Yes, of course. We were not able to get quick fixes for either of the three of our problems. We have always conversed, one on one and together., as children and in their adulthoods. Obviously, not always agreeing, but communicating with our differences and having much peace.

I was questioned about the MS effect and my usual adverse reactions. They had never seen me wanting someone to feel sorry for me, and I never have wanted sorrow or center stage performances. Was that MS? Maybe sometimes I communicated too much and openly with their significant others. Had the MS caused me to become hypocritical and judgmental? How had I acquired such a warped mind set, reliving some things in the past?

One time I was told by one of my sons that I was not needed as a mother with some things. What? I do not know what brought on that idea. The clarification was that I no longer needed to in-put on lots of things. I definitely agreed with that after I got the full understanding of the, "You are no longer needed as a mother" phrase we had a good laugh on that clarity. It would probably help me to get some professional counseling with the MS disease. At first, I was too hurt and really felt a lot of rejection. Had I been put out to pasture after I had been devoted to him his whole life. We talked, were very frank, and on one happy accord. Funny! I do not purposely get into my sons adult lives and businesses. Often as a mother, I do want to know some of their "5 -W's" choices on limited personal subjects. I am very glad that my sons do not need a "mothering hen" considerations.

They are mature capable responsible adults. Are they? Yes. I have my things to deal with. Yes, there is lots of love and respect between us.

I stated that our sons had done somewhat of a flip flop in their behavior demeanors. One lives about thirty-five miles away on one side of Atlanta. He calls several times weekly. He did visit often, when he had a drivers' license. Presently, he still does with his beautiful, great wife as chauffeur and company to us.

Our other son lives about thirty-five miles away, on the opposite direction from his brother in Atlanta. He calls and visits often too. We all always stay in some kind of contact with each other.

MULTIPLE SCLEROSIS, THE HORRENDOUS, NOTORIOUS, UNINVITED, INTRUDER

I have had weird MS thoughts of hearing from them and really hearing either simply ask, "How are you feeling? May I do something for you today?" Those are the contrary low emotional thoughts projected by the MS monster. I do know that my sons and their families are there if I need them. They do call and inquire lovingly about my concerns. That definitely include my acquired adult daughters too.

That MS monster sometimes does effect my sensitivity. It can really take its toll. Its intrusion is no joke. I would like to think that I do not allow the enemy to cause me so much physical and emotional discomforts. But, since I always feel physical discomforts, I question, who is really calling the shots sometimes?

If I were reading this book, I would probably say that this author is too contradictory and wishy washy too. From all of the people (young, old, male, female), I am around at all times, in all occasions, they appear to be genuinely at peace and encouraging to me, and enjoy my company.

I love my family, whether we agree or lovingly disagree sometimes. I guess that makes us as normal as the next family. I do not want to leave my readers with the impression that I am a pompous indecisive person. I want this book to express facets in my life after MS took up its free residence. However, again many other things had to be placed in the picture, in order to make the needed background of the connections to fit my life puzzle together, before and after the MS diagnosis.

I pray for GOD'S healing. I pray for patience in waiting. No weapon formed against me shall prosper. Within, I know that I face and bear painful obstacles physically and emotionally. I try to let go and let GOD. The unfavorable, resurfacing remnants and issues too often crop up. I should really move on and regroup my thoughts. I often do, sadly, until the next time. Unfortunately, those words are easier said than accomplished in lots of situations. I humor myself and find personal peace all of the time through catharsis.

E. C. McCOLLUM-FLANIGAN

EMOTIONAL FEAR / MINOR DEPRESSION

Occasional thoughts of emotional fear surface. Now, I am proud to say that I do not dwell on thoughts of being permanently wheelchair or bed confined. My faith lets me know that GOD allows me to be in control, with this invisible and unpredictable disease, regardless of what others may think. I hope to eliminate most of the moments of depression. Even when I am at my lowest.
I am really able to do that.

EMOTIONAL GUILT

Why should I carry emotional guilt for something that I am not guilty of? Sure, there will be times when I will be slow and hold up the pace of something. I will need assistance, but I will not carry a baggage of guilt. I think that I deal with the MS mood swings very well.

HAPPINESS

I want to be happy. I want everyone to be happy. No, I am not joyous to maybe gain advantages and attentions by being disabled. Those are cheap shots to me.
My shortcoming is that I am not happy when people around me are not happy. I am happy that I live in an area that is endowed with expert medical staff and modern technology facilities to help patients and rehabilitation as presently possible. I can always receive the benefits and keep abreast of updates in the MS field.

SADNESS

Yes, I do have a lot of sad moments. Some of them are self inflicted. So, I can do better through prayer, and when I choose. Most of them come with frustrations to me that others may cause.

Who am I blaming? Anyone who I feel retaliates and intimidates me. That greatly includes when I have said something or did something hurtful to others. I must try to get to the bottom of the discord and make true amends. My sadness will not leave until closure is brought to my shortcoming of the problem.

SHAME

No, I am not ashamed to be the way the MS intruder's attacks brought me down from successful modifications in my lifestyle. For, I know that I am still making success in my life.

COGNITIVE EFFECTS

I have learned to adjust my agenda when needed. I have always, before MS, made "To Do" lists for completing tasks. I have not become forgetful, misplaced, or impatient. I do think about my lack of interest in hobbies I once thoroughly enjoyed completing, then I rationalize and think that," However, I have been there and done that too many times." I really do not care to over indulge in the hobbies as I once did. Those hobbies included completion in a week's time 1000 pieces of jig-saw puzzles, crossword or word find puzzles, amateur painting, playing my piano and guitar, reading a thick novels weekly, consistently daily doing my exercises, sewing or crocheting, organizing and watching photos and home videos, etc.

What has happened? I do not like my lack of interest from my hobbies, but I know that I have to be in the mood to successfully enjoy and complete them. Sometimes now, I will take out and put something in sight so that I will get around to working or playing on it. Then, after a few days, I still have not started a project, not to mention near completion of one. I will then remove whatever it was out, until I will get in the mood at another time. I may then think, "What has happened to my once very interested focus on the things I enjoyed doing? I dislike what defects the devious intruder has caused there. Those were things I enjoyed to the point that I always made time in my daily schedule to work or play with something interesting to me. I did not do them all at the same time, but on any given week, I was involved and completed any three of them. Where do I go from here? I am going to rekindle my interests and take charge. The reality is, sometimes wrong calls are made. By whom? I guess me. So, if it is me, I can definitely get a better grip on things, ASAP!

<u>PSALM 147:</u> Great is our LORD and mighty in power; HIS understanding has no limit.

<u>JOHN 4: 1</u>
Let not your heart be troubled. You are trusting GOD, now trust in me. (the comforter, JESUS CHRIST)

XI. FINANCIAL ADJUSTMENTS

MALACHI 3: 10
Bring the whole tithe into the storehouse, that there might be food in my house...Test me in this says the LORD ALMIGHTY.

Prior to the occupancy of the rude intruder's residency, I had worked for twenty-nine years as a social worker two years, and as a middle school teacher for twenty-seven years.

I had done the two years of social work in the middle 1960's during the Vietnam War Era. My husband and I lived on the West Coast during his military assignment. My clientele consisted of assisting predominantly Oriental deserted military wives and their children. Although, they legally had military privileges and benefits, sometimes and obviously, they and their legal paper works had gotten lost in the cracks, during their transfers. Their spouses had inadequately and illegally done some undercover finagles to mislead Uncle Sam's family benefits. The military takes care of its own.

My job was to help them locate housing, provide them transportation (using my automobile), to physicians, stores, and other necessary errands. Notably, there were language and culture barriers. The bottom line was to get them reconnected to the military, with proper legal papers, of course, so that their military wives and children, housing, medical benefits, English languages classes, and other benefits would be quickly and successfully established.

I do not remember the consequences from the military authority for the irresponsible spouses.

There were consequences from the military authority for the purposely estranged husbands.

With my salary combined with my husband's military salary, we did okay. Later, after military separation and relocation to our home area, the birth of two sons, and completion of my graduate school career change, my husband was the sole financial benefactor.

We were blessed greatly. We did successful things. We endured and solved newly weds' marriage personality and other minor conflicts. Redundantly, by somebody's statistics, we had the American Dream: two children, two vehicles, a tri-leveled house accompanied with a large yard, two dogs, and a very temporary cat. We vacationed yearly and our lives were full of interested activities.

We were situated among both sides of our families. We did not really lack for anything financially. No, we did not have an abundance of money, we spread and used what we had wisely. After over three years of being a full time house mom, I began teaching middle school full time. Yes, I thoroughly enjoyed being a full time house mom with my children. It would take me too long to list all of activities, at home and away from home, bonding we shared. Many a times my sons and I, my sister and her young sons, my other sister's children would spend hours together at Six Flags, the zoo, cultural events, shopping, Bible classes/Vacation Bible School, visiting relatives and friends, concerts, and on and on, etc. Oh yea, sometimes we would just spend time people and plane watching. at Hartsfield Jackson Airport.

Yes, that was during the eras when airports had glass, high story observation decks.

Okay, your are right. What has this got to do with the diagnosis of MS for me?

Well, again, I want to connect and fill in any missing gaps that may questionably appear without closure to some of my statements.

MULTIPLE SCLEROSIS, THE HORRENDOUS, NOTORIOUS, UNINVITED, INTRUDER

Sure, most teachers do not have enormous salaries. We worked together with our salaries to our advantages. We had lots of financial good times and experienced wonderful family adventures.

Fast forwarding along to the years of the MS diagnosis. Redundantly again, for the umpteenth time, I persevered through about two years of physical exams from A to Z. The tests varied from individual physician procedures to specific laboratory blood tests, and hospital out-patient tests.

With all of those tests, the fees were not cheap by no means. I had appointments with the following specialists seeking a diagnosis:

two podiatrists	two chiropractors	one gastroenterologist
three physical therapists	three neurologists	one immunologist
one medical doctor	one aquatic therapist	one neurosurgeon
one urologist	one gynecologist	pharmacists

There were other medical coordinators and liaison staff members that I visited.

Gratefully, my husband's work company provided/s excellent medical benefits that cover eighty percent of the cost, after being verified. The over the counter medications are out of pocket monies. My remaining twenty percent and over the counter costs averages approximately two hundred and fifty dollars monthly.

Something good and helpful happened from applying shared advise from my MS Group friends. I was told about mail order, home delivery, pharmaceutical disbursals. After my husband and I requested information from my husband's insurance coordinator, after receiving the triple prescriptions and triple refills from my neurologist, and after completing all required paper work, I was approved. WOW! What a true blessing.

The medications' mail order saved/s me major financial big bucks. Unfortunately, the most expensive medication can not be approved for mail order delivery form my husband's insurance because syringes are not sent through the mail. That really makes good sense to me, with illegal drug usages so prevalent.

So, each month my intravenous medication supply, cost me approximately two-hundred plus dollars. That amount is included in the pre-stated out of pocket monies dispersals. I can afford that amount from savings on the lesser amount that I spend through the mail order program. Just a phone call, or an internet contact, will update the refills until it is time to see my physician again.

Five years earlier, before the MS's intruding presence, I had planned to retire from teaching after the thirty years requirement for full benefits in my state. There was never any doubts in my mind about taking an early retirement or making another career change. I managed my finances very well. We bought, bought, and bought as I deemed fittingly for my family, especially for our sons.

Today, I buy, buy, and buy for my precious Grandchildren. All of them, my biological ones as well as some of my acquired ones. It does not matter to me. Being different with my biological and immediately acquired ones would sadly matter big time to me. I give lots of gifts to others too. I give/lend money to my young immediate friends when they need a little financial help. I am grateful that the GOOD LORD enables me to do that, without me robbing Peter to pay Paul for my own expenses. Sometimes I receive paybacks. Some times I will not accept paybacks.

One thing I have tried to instill in my sons was the cliché, "A stitch in time saves nine." Sure, they know what that means.

I do not need too many additional material things. I am quite satisfied with what I have.

As for as my tract record for purchasing things, I was/am very slow in buying fad things most of the times. Therefore, I would shop and shop, from mall to mall, or individual stores, no matter what items I was seeking purchases for, until I located what I really desired. I bought good material, expensive name brand items, because I knew that I would probably use them forever. I do not change a lot of things, because they are traditional contemporary good items, whether personal or house items. Most of them, are old, are very useful, and in very good shape presently, because they were/are absolutely my preferences.

When I had to retire, I received enough unused sick leave money to tie me over for four months while waiting to begin receiving my regular monthly disability checks. During those four months, I was okay! With hindsight, after I retired, I realized that maybe I should have taken a few more sick leave days off with my regular salary, just to rest. Unknowingly to me before that time, I would loose about three thousand dollars, that would be taxed back to the state. This statement does not make much logical sense, but trust me, it is true. In other words, one seems to be taxed twice. First, with each monthly federal withholding, and secondly, from the final accumulated lump sum federal withholding. I lost money because I did not use all of my allotted sick leave time. Yes, I took a few days off, but never the maximum allotted days. The real problem was/is, there is a mandatory limited amount of sick leave days that are allowed to be carried over for accumulation through the years. For example, for my twenty-five years of full time teaching, without staying out of school, (who would ever do that any way), I possibly could have accumulated about 275 to 300 sick leave days. Okay, the state's maximum accumulation is 125 days. Now you see what I mean. Many of us teachers wanted to give some days to other teachers who had had to deal with long term illnesses for themselves or some family member. That needed courtesy was never approved by the state, while I taught.

Each year I could have used my sick leave time and saved myself some money. However, I enjoyed what I did. I did not like to leave my students hanging. Yes, there were excellent substitutes.

A dedicated teacher knows that it is more work to be absent that it is to be present.

Another hindsight thing I could have done was to take several months of sick leave the first semester of that up coming school year. Then I could have retired after using most of my accumulated sick leave days. No, I could not have done that even if it had been recommended to me. Why?

It would have really bothered me to know that I had assigned students, and I did not even know who they were, not to mention not being able to actually teach and get to know them just to save some bucks. Wouldn't that be awful? To have a child with a long-term absent full time teacher that they had never met or interacted with. Yes!

I have not let the MS intruder rob me of my flexibility financially. I have a true belief, like I thought of my father, that I will never be broke. Not being broke might mean that I will possess only a very few dollars, but that verifies the fact that I will not be broke. Sure, I had to modify my random spending on some things. Not to the point that I am without owning or goofing off buying junk, when I choose to do so.

Lastly, but really at the top of my budget list, is my obedience to the LORD. I continue to pay my tithes, and give gifts and offerings abundantly. I am proud of me!

In summary, logically, I receive less money from disability than from a regular pay check.

Luckily, I am okay and my bills are in the black too. I also receive a small alternate social security monthly check, that I use for petty cash, and for things that I do not usually need to purchase, but that I purchase anyway. I call it my fun money. In reality, it is also my bills' money.

With the combined incomes of my husband and I, we do just fine. We manage to come and go, travel, and goof out buying things, as we pretty much please to do so. Thank GOD, we are not destitute.

PSALM 37: 3
Trust in the LORD and do good. Then you will live safely in the land and prosper.

PSALM 37: 16
Better the little that the righteous have, than the wealth of many wicked…

XII. SEXUALITY

1ST CORINTHIANS 7: 3 & 4

3) Let the husband render unto the wife due benevolence and likewise also the wife unto the husband.
4) The wife hath not power of her own body, but the husband; and likewise also the husband hath not power of his own body, but the wife.

How does the MS monster effect one's Sexuality?

I have attended a few Multiple Sclerosis seminars and lectures on sexuality. However, I have not had a one on one sharing exchange about sexuality with MS. Obviously, moods and sexualities may also vary from person to person, depending on individual deteriorations. A dominant factor in this is, the high, the medium, and the low sexual activity levels of the MS patient before the enemy's attack. It goes without saying, who would be effected the most. Sexualities fluctuations may or not be effected negatively emotionally or physically. Those effects would depend on to what extents, the body's libido nerves had/have been damaged.

In seminars, reference books, and other helpful materials, making sexual accommodations and modifications are stressed. To me, an understanding communicative significant, makes the different just as it did/does before MS.

Sexuality is an integral part of living and human relations. Recognition of symptoms of numbness and plasticity may actually make a difference. Sexual balance depends on the couple. It did not take MS to make me aware of that. Therefore, we positively manage just fine.

The take over MS intruded slyly invaded my body after menopause. Therefore, it stands to reason statically, that I had passed my sexual prime time peaks of an average person anyway. Yes, I am sure there are exceptions to the so called "mid-life crisis." So, my husband and I are again okay. Well, it is like anything else that happens with the body. One thing may cause very slight dysfunctions in all areas. The MS intruder has lost again. My husband and are most often understand each other.

I surmise, from some of my research on the subject that sexuality is an extra real problem for some couples. Any one who has been diagnosed with MS or any other Central Nervous System dysfunctions may definitely be unresponsive sexually. That is very easy to understand. There are problems with males and females with nerve dysfunctions.

Sometimes, sexuality does not become a problem, because there may be specific sexual nerve damages that an individual has and could care less about, as well as have absolutely little sexual desire. So, when there is no sexual desire, then there is little sexual problem. Thus, there is a real definite problem when a healthy partner has sexual desires, and the other partner has little sexual desires. I know that there are mix-matched couples facing and solving this true life problem.

MS, and other CNS physicians and specific sexual counselors are available to help couples find ways of mending their sexual problems successfully and fulfilling, when there is a need.

XIII. SPIRITUALITY AND MUCH GRATITUDE

PSALM 34:18
The LORD is close to the brokenhearted and saves those who are crushed in spirit.

Without my close relations with JESUS CHRIST, and the fear of GOD, I have no idea of what my mindset would be.

I am so grateful to my LORD and SAVIOR for my active sane being. Sure, sometimes I have asked, after abundantly praying, why has GOD not replaced every diseased cell in my body with healthy cells. Why am I daily trying to be very mindful of consuming beneficial nutrition and other necessary things? Occasionally, I do eat a minimal of junk foods. Why am I conscientiously throughout every day asking GOD to answer my supplications to HIM? Does it mean that I am a hypocrite and lack faith?

No, no, no, I definitely have faith and belief in JESUS CHRIST. What is missing? GOD promised to answer our prayers, especially when we ask for HIS will to be done.

I do realize that I do not see GOD'S big picture. I do realize that GOD'S timing is not like my timing. I do realize that GOD works in mysterious ways. I do realize that GOD'S multiple choice answers are: yes, no, immediately, and wait faithfully.

As pre-stated, I have repeatedly tried modern technology prescriptions, holistic alternative methods, prayers, anointed with blessed oils, open prayer, private prayer in my prayer closet, direct and intercessory prayer.

I definitely know that my healing is coming from my LORD and SAVIOR, JESUS CHRIST.

I feel that GOD is going to use me as a testimonial to other MS patients to keep the faith and graciously let me tell the world that there is Devine healing.

PROVERBS 16:1

We can make our plans, but the final outcome is in GOD'S hands.

Fill me, joy of JESUS anxiety shall cease And heaven's serenity be mine JESUS bring me peace.

XIV. FAMILY—LOVING GRAND CHILDREN— CHURCH FRIENDS SOCIAL FRIENDS MULTIPLE SCLEROSIS SUPPORT GROUP

1ST JOHN 4:7

Dear friends, let us love one another, for love comes from GOD.

FAMILY

Like any family, we share various interests in our lives. I have a wonderful extended biological and acquired in-laws caring family. I have lots of family members on both sides.

Generations are constantly reproducing. Even though most of my relatives an in-laws reside in the same metro area, that is not to say that a lot of family resides in other states as well.

I do not know all of the youngest generations.

Sure, there are reunions, weddings, funerals, birthday-get-togethers, and all kinds of celebrations, for almost any thought of occasions. Yet, I am still unfamiliar with a lot of young fourth and fifth generations. Atlanta has a humongous Metropolitan area. My family is supportive. Different members are basically concerned, and others periodically inquire about my well being. Of course, some give unbeknown insensitive advise. Some are also full of could have, should have, and would have for the whole "5 W's."

On occasions I have been told that I ask too many questions about things. Maybe I do, but I know that I use inquiry tact. I do not blurt out trying to get in others private concerns. I am not about "he said and she said" gossip and rumors. In spite of being somewhat cut down and told that I sometimes ask too many questions, I have yet to see those same persons walk away from listening to the replies when they want to know the answer to what I have asked someone. I like to know the truth from the source whenever possible.

Some relatives and acquaintances are satisfied by believing what they have heard through the grape vine about this MS intruder's break-in. I can rationalize for them. I may have not communicated with them in years, so they too, may not feel confident enough to call or approach me to receive the factual information from the horse's mouth from yours truly.

I have been guilty of that kind of long range information concerning some of my relatives too. Therefore, I do not hold any type of resentments or grudges from others. When I experience hearing news about others, I too, rationalize and feel that the person who had informed me about what had/is happening to a relative or friend, was/is in a close position to relate the most current update, regression and progression on the relative in question. So, I too, procrastinate in making direct contact with some relatives from time to time also.

I am okay when experiencing the third degrees. It is somewhat easier when I share about my condition and know that there is an understanding, and true inquisitive conversation with others.

I am somewhat hurt when questions about MS are explained to the best of my knowledge, and then I receive negative feedback. True, I do get sensitive from this supremely unwanted MS intruder. However, I have concluded that my sensitivity is only bad and tearful when comments were/are ignorantly misinterpreted or related untruthfully, and generally stated that I am the cause and blame for this MS catastrophe. How can I be the cause and effect of this monster?

MULTIPLE SCLEROSIS, THE HORRENDOUS, NOTORIOUS, UNINVITED, INTRUDER

My relatives are super, but again some of them are hard-core and somewhat disrespectful of others opinions, simply because they think that they are always right about everything. Most every one knows that that is a humanistic impossibility. However, is not that an occasional unrealistic style for some people anyway? It does bother me when someone wants to incorrectly shove his or her misguided ideals and warped opinions shoved down someone else's throats. So, maybe I am judgmental about that default too. Again, it is somewhat normal in any family, dysfunctional or not, for some members to agree when they disagree all over the world. Why? Many reasons. Usually when that happens to me, I just say that I am sorry, I made another mistake, and move on, because they probably will not see anything another way any way. I know, and I know that I have over stated about not respecting others opinions to the hilt. Frankly, I do tend to run that opinion thing in the ground in my thoughts. Why is that so important to me, before and after the MS monster slid in and illegally took residence. I do not know. Whose "couch" do I need to be on?

There were a few times after being diagnosed, I had slight self-pity thoughts of being neglected by my many nephews and nieces. Some of them do visit and call, just to say hello. "How are you feeling, do you need any help?" I estimate that I have approximately forty first generation biological and in-law nieces and nephews living in the Metro area. Do I blame them? Absolutely not, because I lovingly and definitely do the same thing in reverse.

Of course, when we see each other, we are very cordial. We will exchange, "How are you doing" greetings. We usually hug each other. I was pretty close to most of them when they were young children and teenagers. Some of them moved farther away when they became adults.

Most of them married. Most of them also divorced at some points. Most of the divorced ones, have remarried or have other significant others. We always are happy to run into each other in the streets somewhere. I do tell them to call or visit me anytime, and I may do the same in return.

But, do you know what? The honest answer came to me quickly. I am guilty of the same thing. Presently, I have only one maternal aunt living. I visit and call her periodically. Yet, I do admit that I do fail to call or visit her as much as I should. Therefore, a pot can not call a kettle black. Since beginning this book, one other loving maternal aunt has passed. I also have two paternal aunts living, (My father's brothers wives.) Notably, on my husband's side of his family, he has several aunts living. Therefore, I too, honor and recognize them as my aunts. One of them also has passed while writing this book.

To my knowledge, there are no unsolved grudges or discord family feuds. If there were, I am sure that I would know a little something about them. I am blessed because I know that if I really needed anything possible, some one in my, family would try to supply my every need to help me and shower me with love, attention, and support. I love them dearly too! They may say something negative about it, but that would be okay with me too. I would show my appreciation.

My family respects my MS independency. They know that I want to use my capabilities without interferences. My family respects my abilities to do what I can, enjoy things, and complete all of my little projects when I am in the moods to do so. Sometimes, my very close family members, some one may relate to me, what I need to do, or what I should not be doing.

I feel like they know that when I really need physical and emotional boosts, I know that they are there/here for me.

They also know that I do not ask favors, just to seek attention. I have always, and I still ask them to attend complimentary and enlightening programs with me. They know that they may tell me no, because of their lack of interests, and I will respect their refusals. It is not like, and I thank GOD, that, "I can not attend, if you will not go with me."

We share our love, even though I do not hear from most of them, on a regular basis. Many of my relatives will drive by my house and 'honk' saying hello. That is somewhat okay with me, because, I am still a low-key person, before and living with the indwelling, enemy MS intruder. The enemy is sly and strong, but it is also somewhat of a coward knowing to be in hiding at certain times. Yes, I know it is always within, but it knows that I know that it is also psychotic, sneaking and hiding, waiting on its silent notorious planned secret attacks.

LOVING GRAND CHILDREN

During the period that I was going through all types of tests, seeking a diagnosis for the horrible physical ailments, my precious second grandson was born. He was/is just too cute and cuddly.

The MS enemy messed with me there. I did conquer its scheming though. Because my balance was so off, I did not take chances walking around carrying him. I did not want to drop him. Consequently, that is the only reason that I do not carry any young infants. I just love them.

I hold them, after someone else has handed them to me. I cuddle and play with them.

Remember my husband and I have acquired approximately fifteen or twenty non-biological related loving grandchildren. Sometimes, we take some of them on our "mini-field trips", church programs, family gatherings, mini-shopping, out to lunch or dinner, visit our home with or without their parents, etc., and on and on. For those loving reasons, that is how I did win the MS enemy's anti-child loving game. I held, cuddled, and loved them in every way, but carrying the one who could not walk at the time. WOW!

Later on, when my second grandson learned to walk, he, as well as all of the other grandchildren, always stayed/stay in my home on periodic intervals of weeks with my husband and me. Today, that is our special bonding pattern. We visit the Grands. The Grands visit us.

The Grands spend parts of their school, and summer vacations with us. I am quite able to take care of them. You should see and visit us at Christmas.

So, MS monster, you failed, so tuck your tail and leave!

We do all kinds of multi-fun in door and outside activities. We attend church, go to parks, fun pizza parties, put-put, video game arcades, eating out in nice restaurants and fast food, special plays, to the mountains, to the man made beaches, amusement parks, in and out of state, and attend sports activities, etc, on and on. Many times their parents go along with us as chaperones and over all family bondings. We do lots of paper, coloring, and cutting, artsy crafty activities. They know the rule of cleaning up all of their mess. Some times we overlook some of the minute cleaning until later. However, it is stressed to them not to leave junk in the floor or areas of the house that may cause me to trip and fall. They have seen me trip and fall many times to know exactly why that precaution is taken. They are wonderful in helping me get up when I fall, or consoling me when I cry.

We watch juvenile movies. I take them to visit local young playmates/relatives in my area.

We also have a friend who takes them on outings with him and his children. This past summer he took them to the Atlanta Zoo, a rare and real Drive-in Movie, and out to eat and play. We play various board games and puzzles., video games, etc. They play around on the computer. They use the internet, only when I monitor their choice of programs and web sites. They know that my husband and I do not listen to negative hip-hop music or watch clad dressed persons in movies. They know that they do not do the same when they are with us. Okay, one may think, well, that leaves very little for them to listen to and watch on the media. You are correct. But, that's what we do, and they know what channels to watch.

I have my way of shopping with them. Not mall shopping, except at Christmas times and other holidays. We enjoy a mall's decorations and Merry, Merry, Ho, Ho, Ho's. We have driven through the local and famous, "Lights of the Season" exhibits.

I do take them shopping in the biggest department stores with Granddaddy along. The older ones take terms pushing me in my wheelchair. Yes, the MS intruder knows that I am unable to walk for long periods. Very seldom do I shop with them all together. I push the younger ones in the store's shopping cot. We have lots of fun together, and also with my husband. The biggest problem is, I become a sucker, like with their parents. No, they do not do much whining and pleading for things. They basically know what I will buy

MULTIPLE SCLEROSIS, THE HORRENDOUS, NOTORIOUS, UNINVITED, INTRUDER

usually, but not binding, before we enter the stores. They have selective choices of what I purchase for them.

I jokingly rationalize and I do mean it, and say that, "I did not have a grandmother, to acquire a grandmother's role model." Therefore, I make my own rules as I go along. Yes, they are moral, good mannered, most of the times, a little normal aggravating, respectful, and obedient rules.

They are precious and special little people to me. They are helpful in during small chores when they are vacationing with us. Our daily agendas stay full. That's our choice.

We share some wonderful good times and adventures. Then, it is time for them to return to their homes, until the next time.

The house becomes so empty sounding. After the Grands leave, we will clean the house in the ways that we like it to be, until the next time. We really miss them. However, we would not want it to be any other way. We love them, we nuture them, and we spoil them and send them home until our visits to them, or their visits to us.

The older ones live about twenty-five minutes away from us. They are always coming and going, spending a few days with us, especially when there are special family and church functions. Also, they are with us very often when there is not anything going on. We have a great relationship with their mother and their other siblings. We consider her one of our girls too.

Two of the Grands in Atlanta, and two of the Grands from Florida have attended MS seminars, MS fun days, and several MS functions with us. They have heard medical explanations and have seen medical visuals from several neurologists speakers in Atlanta. They have been polite to other MS patients they have seen with canes, crutches, wheelchairs, scooters, etc. They have received MS pamphlet explaining MS from a child's point of understanding. They have gone to physical therapy sessions with me. They have very good companionship for helping me get around and carrying things. There is so much inner and overt love among us. WOW!

My husband and I keep the grandchildren dream alive. We attend some of their school functions in state and out of state yearly. We give them petty spending cash. They voluntarily add to their spending cash by cleaning up around our house or in the yard, then stating how much they need to be paid for their jobs. Funny, but we do in reasonable amounts. We thoroughly enjoy them and most of their tricks.

The horrendous MS monster, does not beat them with his cruel effects. They win with me.

CHURCH FAMILY FRIENDS

My paternal family and a lot my husband's maternal and paternal family have always had the same community church membership until some of the family members changed their church memberships upon adulthoods.

At, some time, in past decades, I remember well, when my Church's membership was primarily and dominantly biologically related. That ancestral membership congregation was very common, and still is sometimes and in some geographical locations, because there were paternal and maternal community descendants.

No, no, no, and definitely not the results of incestral relationships. This may seem to appear as an untruth to people who have never, ever lived in a small town. However, people who have common backgrounds, will know exactly what I am saying and know that incest was not an option or result of the family relationships.

I will briefly give an example of how the relationships have come to be in the past.

This background is not MS, but it plays a role in my Family, Friends, and MS Support Group positively to enhance the whole me.

Okay, please follow me. There were/are several children in one family. There were/are several children in other families. Neither of the families were/are biologically related. They just reside in the same locality. Thus, as the children from the opposite families criss-cross and become married, their children will be double, and in a lot of cases triple relatives. A clearer example is when sisters or brothers marry other sisters and brothers in each other families. Obviously their children will be biologically double relatives in the same family. That absolutely, and definitely result in no manners of incest.

MULTIPLE SCLEROSIS, THE HORRENDOUS, NOTORIOUS, UNINVITED, INTRUDER

That is what happens in small populated areas. Dating and marriage choices become slim among residents in the small town population. Trust me, when people date among a small town population, oral or recorded family history is researched, just to avoid inter-related datings and marriages. Rarely, but every once in a while, related persons will marry.

My Church Family's motto is, "The Church where Love abounds!"

Members and visitors greet, hug, pray, sing, shout, communicate, share great compassion, and dance for JESUS. The most important thing we do is receive and obey GOD'S WORDS.

We know, whether, it is abided by or ignored, JESUS CHRIST, is our LORD and SAVIOR.

Being spiritually saved and born again is the main focus. Other things and needs will be supplied under that umbrella. My Pastor is an excellent, wonderful, and Spirit-filled, praying Shepherd!

I have read the BIBLE three or four times, in varied editions. I have read THE KING JAMES AND THE LIVING, NO, NO, NO, and of course NOT, I definitely do not profess to understand or interpret much of the whole WORD. I try to and must have my personal BIBICAL and meditation time daily. I have to ask, seek, and knock for peace daily. I pray, not only for me, I must pray for others as well as for the world. I appreciate my LORD'S goodness and mercy to all.

MULTIPLE SCLEROSIS SUPPORT GROUP

I had been diagnosed about two years before I actively got involved with a local MS Support Group. I wanted to become a part of a group. I checked out the meetings schedules in the metro area, but unfortunately the meetings were not in my close vicinity and were scheduled for night meetings. No, I was not afraid to attend one at night. I simply kept making excuses and did not attend the meetings.

I received lots of information from the National and Local MS Societies. I think that my name and address were on the data bases from my previous hospital stay. Therefore, I decided that I would treat myself to one of the seminars at a conference center in Atlanta. There was really no reason for me not to attend, because the meetings were only short distances away from my residence. That one meeting attendance got me started. Presently, I attend all kinds of MS Programs.

The Main Local Society has guest physicians that specialize in MS. I have listened to testimonies from MS patients, as well as some famous media testimonies and presentations.

At one meeting, I saw some acquaintances that I had met earlier at an MS Seminar.

One of the guys stated that he wanted to initiate an MS Support Group on another specific side of the metro. I discovered that we live in the same town. Fortunately, working together, with a few other local acquaintances, thus the new group was formed.

We meet monthly. We share our concerns and lots of common experiences. We chit-chat regularly because we are just a phone call away from each other. The Group has had excellent speakers, show and tell experts in physical therapy, nutrition, the disease modifying immune system drugs…

"A, B, C, R", injections representatives, and other needed concerns and topics. "A B C R" is the common lingo for the disease modifying intravenous drugs of Avonex, Betaseron, Capoxone, and Rebif. Another prescription used drug is Novantrone.

I learned about the advantages and low cost factors of pharmaceutical home delivery.

Wow! That was excellent information for me. We share and exchange pros and cons, side effects, common emotional ups and downs., as well as of the "A B C R" medications.

The Group is small, caring, and growing in numbers. There are males and females in attendance. The average age is approximately forty. I was/am glad to communicate and identify with other "People of Color" close to my age. Yes, the Group has younger ages and other races.

Caregivers often attend, including my husband.

I can identify with ex-public school educators. They too retired from the classroom because of lessened mobility. We come from varied professions. Some members of the Group are still working.

Some members are medically retired, Some members are seeking limited employment. Several months ago, I heard a new comer introduce herself and stated where she resided. Bingo! We live in the same town. Since then we have attended meetings, conferences, visited each others homes, met family members, and shared our MS ups and downs. I need that common compatible friendship. No matter where we go, she always says that she likes to drive at her cost. I enjoy the rides and conversations. I really like every member of the Group. No, there is no favoritism. We are all glad to share with someone who has been attacked by the MS enemy. No, we do not want anyone to be attacked. It is wonderful to be able to share common experiences.

Our sharings include subjects about diagnoses, medications, physicians, and insurance, our strengths and weaknesses, as well as our families. We also share subjects concerning employment, retirement, mobility, transportation, organ dysfunctions caused by the MS monster, etc, as well as the emotional roller coaster dilemmas.

Presently, the Group has not been openly candid about sexuality, embarrassing bowel problems, and a few embarrassing other experiences the MS intruder has invaded us with.

We will get secure and comfortable enough to share those things openly soon.

Some of us will soon become one on one sharing exchange partners.

We do attend Local Seminars where we hear intimate topics from physicians and MS advocates. We hear lectures with visual aids, questions and answer sessions, multiple free informational books, gadgets, demonstrations, samples, and all kinds of hand-outs.

Sometimes free examinations covering weight, diabetics, blood pressure tests, bone density screenings, etc. We have heard from a few professional sports persons who have been diagnosed or has a close relative with MS. We are always served refreshments and nutritious lunches or buffets.

The auto parking is always free too, and that is a plus in down town Atlanta.

I like associating with my friends and caregivers in the Group. I plan to attend two other larger Groups. Presently, and by the time this is read, I will have attended many MS functions.

As an example of a typical MS Seminar or sponsored Program, one was entitled "Interactive Multiple Sclerosis Education Day."

The Program included:

1) Improving Function Through Rehabilitation
2) The Future of Multiple Sclerosis Research
3) Multiple Sclerosis Encouragement

There will also be available interactive demonstrations, physical therapy demonstrations, MS aquatic class demonstrations, home exercise balance exercises, and occupational tips, etc.

Sometimes I choose to participate in pre-scheduled teleconferences. When I am interested in the teleconference subjects, registration is just a phone call away.

Redundantly, again, I am fortunate enough to have access to unlimited MS medical professionals help and shared knowledge. I feel sadly for persons diagnosed with MS, or any CNS disease and their families, who do not receive all of modern technology, researched and approved medications, information, and support to help comfort them physically and emotionally through the devastations and deteriorations that occur. May GOD bless them as HE does and let HIS will be done.

JOHN 15: 12 & 13

12) This is my commandment, that ye love one another, as I have loved you.
13) Greater love hath no man than this, than a man lay down his life for his friends.

XV. PESSIMISTIC VERSUS OPTIMISTIC REALITIES

<u>PSALM 25: 15</u> My eyes are always looking to the LORD for HE alone can rescue me from the traps of my enemies.

I remember seeing a poster from somewhere at sometime that stated:
"AN OPTIMIST SEES AN OPPORTUNITY
IN EVERY PROBLEM.
A PESSIMIST SEES A PROBLEM IN
EVERY OPPORTUNITY."

One may alter his/her life by altering the circumstances to advantages.

Negative emotions and doubts can overflow in any person, especially those diagnosed with MS. Why? Basically, I feel that the disease is one of the most deteriorating, non- restorative diagnosed diseases existing. Quite often, 'the light in the tunnel' is invisible.

Again, examples of very frequently asked questions include;
"What is going to eventually happen to you"
"Will I ever feel better and not miserable?"
"What is the point in trying to do anything…?"

Trust me, a problem can be found very easily with the MS dwelling within, invisibly leaving its damages. Remaining up-beat is a tremendous day to day task. It often takes only one little questionable comment from someone, for me to become sensitive big time. If the comment jogged my memory of something that was unpleasant in the past, I may become a temporary basket case. No, no, I do not want any one's self pity. Over sensitiveness is a main move in the MS intruder's strategy game play.

Remember, an optimistic sees opportunities. I know that I am suppose to find something good, no matter how minute, it may be, in every situation. However, "to thine own self be true." Unfortunately, for me, I often harbor reservations and the lack of joy in finding opportunities, mentally and physically for feeling bad in some part of my body all of the time.

Yes, I do know that it is not GODLY, to not experience joys and trials in life's sufferings.

I remind myself not to be so sensitive and vulnerable due to the insecurities and survival skills I must handle daily. I am so grateful that GOD allows me to possess those positive skills of maintenance. No, I am not an ingrate. I know where I have come from. I know how I went down, from busy, planned, and regular spur of the moment daily agendas changes, to becoming a person who was unable to personally or independently function for a short period. I thank my unconditional SAVIOR for blessing me to get back up. As a very popular contemporary gospel song is titled. "We Fall Down, but We Get Up." Personal, factual, optimism is forever worth my gratification and praises to HIM.

Obviously, with the notorious indwelling MS, I am not one-hundred percent healthy. But, I am blessed and grateful that I am able to do pretty much what I want to do. Needless to say, in reality, who is? Fortunately, I am definitely and positively not, nor will I become one-hundred per -cent disabled either. I have this comforting inner feeling that GOD is using me through these trials and tribulations as a testimony to others, and to me to keep on holding on to HIM.

Redundantly again, presently, I am not able to hop, run, or jump. But, most of all, I am very mobile for self preservation. I am quite capable of driving my vehicle anywhere I want to go. I can maintain my home, cook meals, do daily exercises other things, in reason that I choose to do. Sure, I listen to my body. I stop and rest when my body tells me to do so. Normally, after about a maximum of forty-five minutes of standing, walking, (with cane) or during any kind of chore, the extra 'tired and loosing my energy' feelings in my feet and legs let me know that it is really time to rest. I then sit or lie down for about fifteen minutes and let my personal brain computer processor reactivates and recuperate. I am obedient to my body, no matter what I am involved in.

I do get a little apprehensive when I get "the real tired on my feet feeling", in a public place and there is absolutely no place to sit for a few minutes. I know from experience, that I am very subject to falling on the spot. My optimal goal is to avoid falling down and causing more nerve damage. So, what do I do in those situations? I quickly look around and sit on stacked supportive boxes, shelves, counters, or an unoccupied store's manual or electric wheelchair, etc. Most places have at least one accommodating place to sit. I have asked a store employee to please fine me a seat for a few minutes.

That request has always been granted. I think that being seen using a cane is the password.

I do reiterate that, loving companions, associates, and even strangers assist me when they see my needs. Never do I have to worry about carrying or dropping items in stores and restaurants. By my using a cane, some help will be offered. Being optimistic, the good parts include when physically I am unable to maneuver as I would like to move around, and doing what I once took for granted, usually some one will come to my rescue and inquire if I need some help.

GOD is good through others' assistances. There are good caring moral people among us, in spite of lots of evil and lewdness we see in the media.

Sometimes when I mini-shop solo, whoever is in charge at the facilities, (sales clerks, waitresses, flight attendances, ushers, etc.) offer their personal assistance when they observe the need. Most of the time I use a manual shopping cart in lieu of any store's motorized wheelchair, or my cane, whether I am alone or with someone. Pushing and lending on a shopping cart is the only way I feel secure to browse or shop. I substitute the walking leaning on a shopping cart for my treadmill exercise.

Yes, to me, I am usually an optimist. I must say that there have been a few times when some family member has stated to me that my interpretation of what they had stated was way off. How? Well, they should not have been playing one of their poor communicating guessing games.

. I only get on a pity-pot and think that I am a burden and insecure, only when I allow negative pessimistic feelings of this MS intruder to entice me into those emotions. I pray and those insecure thoughts disappear very quickly. This intruder ought to be smart enough to soon realize that it is definitely not going to be experiencing a hospitality vacation or compassionate dwelling within me.

Optimistically, I am a very superior, rude, and hostage landlord to the MS dweller. I do not have any guilt or remorse in my rudeness and bad manners to this MS enemy trying to live rent free within.

PHILLIPIANS 4: 11
…GOD'S peace will guard your hearts and minds as you live in CHRIST JESUS.

XVI. THE PRESENT AND LIFE STYLE CHANGES

PSALM 143: 8
Let the morning bring me word of YOUR unfailing love, for I have put my trust in YOU. Show me the way I should go, for to YOU I lift up my soul.

    To my best recall, it has been about eight years, in hindsight, that I will say that the MS intruder began its entrance in my life. Prior to that time, I did not have any temporary sickness that I did not recover from in a short time.
    Since the uninvited and unwelcome intruder's diagnosis, I have learned how to listen to my body, pace my activities, and rest quickly when I get tired of whatever thing I was/am involved.
    I guard my off-balanced condition by using my cane, or by holding on to strong stationery objects while walking. I walk as freely and independently most of the times in my home. However, in my house and everywhere I go that have steps, or slopes, I have to always hold the banisters. I am unable to ascend or descend without tripping or falling without holding the banisters.
    I try to keep active everyday. Recently, for no particular reason, I have gotten lazy with my exercise routine. I have skipped my twice weekly aquatic exercises. I have also been off schedule riding my stationery bicycle and walking on my treadmill. I have no excuse,

especially because I have all of the time in the world to participate in those activities for my advantages. I know to continuously follow through with treatments and exercises to lessen attacks. Trust me though, I will be back on my exercise regimen before this book is published.

I have really gotten use to not working. As much as I liked teaching, after getting a grip on this Sabbatical, I can not think of being in a classroom now, unless I am visiting one. I hear positive things about teachers, students, and the whole educational processes that must happen for successful education requirements and accomplishments. But, I do not wish that I was in a classroom with the negative things and disruptive behaviors, paper work, meetings, etc. Sure, I experienced negative things and behaviors, but I was in a positive mind set because I knew that those things happened in the real world of teaching. However, I have gotten a break from those things, so I am okay. I give honor and respect to the majority of the well-behaved and successful academic students. I hope that the opposites will turn their lives and school days into successes also.

I attend my now, tri-annual physical appointments to my neurologist. Of course, if there is a need at anytime, I shall make an appointment to go to him. I daily take my proper medications, I am trying my best to remain stabilized with my present mobility, and I will continue to be mobile.

I still have things to do and places to go.

There is an aggravating occurrence that somehow seems to periodically happen to my disadvantage. I try to place my feet firmly and carefully everywhere I walk. Sadly to say, in spite of trying to avoid miss-stepping, I will slip, usually on a step, trip, usually by not holding my toes upward while walking, twist my ankle, or bump a foot or leg, on some object in my pathway.

Yes, they are minor things, but to me, and the MS enemy's influence, they seem somewhat major when soreness occurs from the off balanced tripping or step. The soreness can really cause me to be off balance for a day or two. Then I am in further remittantly recuperation off and on from those minor twists or bumps. It seems somewhat major to me because I am already stumbling around off-balanced. I have had many bruises from the missteps and falls. But, with the MS impairments of the nerves and muscles in my feet, almost any type of injury will cause the blood vessels to become bruised. It usually takes a few weeks to completely heal. I soak the injuries, take ibuprophen, and sometimes pre-scribed anti-bodies when there are open nicks and scratches. I also sometimes take over-the-counter pain medications. I also have occasions when I apply heat and cold to the elevated wounds. I may wear an ace bandage for a short time off and on. Gratefully, I am able to continue moving right along. Again, it seems like Murphy's Law is at work with my clumsiness due to the MS intruder's devious games. Contrary to what I call the MS crook, it is definitely not a game or false. Unfortunately, it is for real. I really try not to take chances, and I try consistently to be very careful. Okay, what is the problem then, with all of the twists, bumps, and turns? The MS enemy, of course, knows how to locate the vulnerabilities in ones life.

MS has clipped a lot of my boundaries in certain ways. For example, I am unable to physically participate in active play with my loving grand children. I am unable to climb mountains, swim well, sun bathe, stroll in the mall, run and jump playing ring game, bowl, and on and on…

But, do you know what? I can do a lot of fun things with them, and my family and acquaintances.

I can read, ride, play while sitting, and watch them play in arcades. I pray and sing with them.

I go to church with them. I kiss, hug, and love them. I watch them play on my piano and guitar.

We always paint, color, cook with them, and find interesting things to lollygag together doing all of the time. Thus, I am able to positively move on, and let the MS intruder know that with or without its boundary clippings, My GOD keeps me in control and successfully moving forward right along.

My present emotional times are manageable. I still get very sensitive some times. The lowest, but for short periods of feeling inadequate, I have had short recurring thoughts that maybe I am becoming a burden and causing problems for others. That feeling may occur when something I had said, in which was a general conversation reply or suggestion to something, was definitely misinterpreted from my meanings.

I still tend to get hurt feelings when I am put in a conversational position to try to figure out the missing pieces of others inadequate, guessing game conversations. Yes, you are right. When sharings and talks are not sensible and complete, they are not decent conversational pieces anyway. Whose fault is that? Everyone, including me, who is involved in those lop-sided so-called conversations, missing information, lop-sided talks.

Yes, I do get over them, until the next time. Just think, all anyone really needs to do is respect each others opinions and agree to disagree. I try to express myself when I experience hurt feelings. I always want to hear the other side of what is going on too. I have to try to get to the real problem, if there is one. Prayer, and openness of the problems are the only ways for me to get to a resolution. Yes, I can do that. Sometimes it just happens a little slowly.

My family and I are close. As some people may categorize about my generation of children, their cousins, and their friends, in my area, "They are still mature spoiled adults." With most of the close parents of adult children, that I know in my area, that was not an intentional, parental short-coming negligent parenting skill. We simply did what we thought we should do. Yes, on occasions it did make some slightly temporary irresponsibility adults. Maybe, that was a definite small town, over-lapping, unrealized way of rearing our off springs. We loved it. Praises to GOD, our adult children really do know the mature, responsible, and Christian things to do. I think that our parents reared us that way too.

Now, here is an up-dated chapter in my present life style.

Presently, unfortunately, my younger son is now divorced. I hate that he and my loving ex-daughter-in-law were unable to mend their issues and remain as one unit with their beautiful children. We will always be in contact with each other along with the Grand children. Regardless of the divorce, she will always be known to me as my daughter-in-law for family recognition and clarity with love.

My older son has gotten married. They had a beautiful little wedding. I love my new daughter-in-law dearly too. She really takes care of my son in ways more than I could put on paper. She too, is a beautiful, compassionate enhancement to our family. I had not expected that the divorce and new marriage would occur thirty-three days apart. I pray for both to have peace and happiness no matter what.

I tend to get very close to my "acquired daughters," including the mother of my older grandson. No, I am not into the ignorant lingo of relating to someone's "Baby's Mama." How low could I go?

In relating in this "Present Me Chapter," I did not biologically have any girls. I feel that I have and presently do, fill in a lot of the gaps, for the lovingly acquired adult females through my sons that are extremely and lovingly in my heart. Being close to all three, I think that I have/do experience some of what any mother of adult females go through. No, I do not like for them to bear pains and trials. I am glad that I can offer my help when it is needed. So, I have shared, and presently share, some adult female (daughters) experiences through them. Of course, I have nieces that I bond with too.

Redundantly, I will cry, when things do not go according to the ways I think maybe they should go. No, I am not a selfish dominating person. No, I do not want things to go my chosen way all of the time. I write my feelings down, then trash the papers later, then I try to move on. Unfortunately, I do remember and compare some aspects of experienced sad times that still may get me in a mood I care and choose to remain in. Why? No, I do not want to save stamps of hurtful times. I am trying to reserve and enjoy the wonderful moments at hand.

Presently, I basically do whatever I choose to do. I cherish the memories of my one hundred percent of past physical endurances. I know how to enjoy life's ups and downs on an even plain most of the times. I am enjoying coming and going to whatever strikes my fancy. I do not drive or fly out of state alone. The MS enemy has not gained any points there because, I travel with my husband all of the times any way.

Yes, the unexplainable, miserable MS intruder, has obviously caused some changes in my life style. The "Present Me and Life Style Changes", will do what has to be done for all of the well-rounded entities and successful things in my life.

I continue praying, learning, adapting, associating, and living at large against the MS enemy. I hope that others who have also experienced the MS intruder's bazaar and devious acts are sincerely capable of positively progressing also. I "THANK YA'LL" for the catharsis healing that I am receiving through writing this book. I know that I have accepted the fact that although I am unable to do what I once physically was capable of experiencing, I have made great compatible accommodations. Sometimes through blood, (from cuts in skin from falling), sweat, and tears, I have let the MS intruder know that it is very hard, but I am a survivor. Perhaps, in the near future, I will become a Multiple Sclerosis Advocate, especially to those in my age bracket.

<u>PSALM 145:2</u> Every day I will praise YOU and extol YOUR name forever and ever.

MULTIPLE SCLEROSIS, THE HORRENDOUS, NOTORIOUS,
UNINVITED, INTRUDER

XVII. CLOSING POEM

There is the horrendous MS intruder
Who loves to become ruder and ruder.
Its confusing and retaliating goal is to win
Its enemy plays are full of sin.

The enemy is definitely sneaky
It loves to make anyone look freaky.
Failures, it hates to admit
It's too obnoxious and cares not to quit.

Life goes on, with changes regard-less
To conquer all of the MS mess.
It is rough, it is tough, it is very aggravating,
Without defeat, life is successfully, escalating.

Lots of challenging trials, and lots of fun times
Excellent supporters to help out in many binds.
What a blessing to always have their love and care
No matter what the circumstances, they are there.

So, MOVE OVER, you monstrous notorious MS
Just face your failure, and get out of the way.
Can't you see, what survivors we are,
We meet our life style goals, every day!

E. C. McCOLLUM-FLANIGAN

Thanks to the DEVINE HEALER,
JESUS CHRIST, our LORD and SAVIOR!

E. C. Mc-FLANIGAN

CREDITS

SCRIPTURES
  HOLY BIBLE PLT PARALLEL EDITION
    King James Version and The Living Bible

  NEW TESTAMENT WITH PSALMS AND PROVERBS
    New Living Translation, 1996
    Tyndale Charitable Trust
    House Publications, Inc.
    Wheaton, Illinois

  THE HOLY BIBLE, KING JAMES VERSION

  WOMEN'S DEVOTIONAL BIBLE
    International Version
    Zondervan Publishing House
    Grand Rapids, Michigan, 1973

JOURNALS...
  NATIONAL MULTIPLE SCLEROSIS SOCIETY
    (a few choice paraphrased information)
    @ 1-800-FIGHT_MS

E. C. McCOLLUM-FLANIGAN

    POETRY. COM
        The International Library of Poetry
        Owings Mills, MD 21117-6282
        E C Mc-Flan (personal copyrighted poem)

    SPINAL COLUMN
        The Magazine of Shepherd Center
        A Specialty Hospital
        Shepherd Center, Inc.
        Atlanta, GA 30309-1465

    UNITED METHODIST HYMNAL
        "Heal Me Hands Of JESUS", by MICHAEL PERRY

    MARLON VINSON FLANIGAN, JOURNALIST / ADVISOR

MULTIPLE SCLEROSIS, THE HORRENDOUS, NOTORIOUS, UNINVITED…INTRUDER,

WILL DEFINITELY BECOME A COMPASSIONATE, INFORMATIONAL, AND AN INSPIRATIONAL, "I CAN'T STOP READING" BOOK FOR INDIVIDUALS, FAMILY MEMBERS, ACQUAINTANCES, AND THEIR CAREGIVERS, WHO KNOW SUFFERERS WITH THE DIBILITATING DISEASE OF MULTIPLE SCLEROSIS.

THIS BOOK REITERATES THAT PRESENTLY, THERE IS NOT AN EXACT CAUSE OR CURE FOR THE DISEASE, IN SPITE OF ITS DEVASTATIONS TO APPROXIMATELY 350,000 PERSONS AFFECTED WITH THE CENTRAL NERVOUS SYSTEM DISEASE.

THE AUTHOR SHARES SOME PERSONAL EMBARRASSING EXPERIENCES, SOME ADAPTIONS TO THE NEGATIVES OF THE DISEASE, AND HER EFFORTS IN KEEPING HER INDEPENDENCE WITH THE DISEASE IN ORDER TO LET OTHER SUFFERERS KNOW THAT THEY ARE NOT ALONE AND CAN MAKE IT.

ABOUT THE AUTHOR

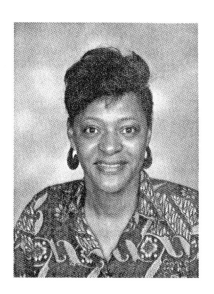

    This non-fiction will definitely become a compassionate, informational, and an inspirational, "I can not stop reading" book for all individuals; including professionals, family members, caregivers, and acquaintances, etc., who know or desire to know sufferers with the debilitating disease of Multiple Sclerosis.

    The book reiterates that presently, there is not an exact cause or cure for the disease, in spite of its devastations to approximately 350,000 persons affected with the disease.

The author shares some personal embarrassing experiences, some adaptations to change the negatives into positives in order to maintain her independence. Personal reflections are shared with the aim of letting other sufferers know that they are not surviving with the catastrophic disease alone.

Corresponding Biblical verses are coordinated throughout the book.

EULA CARLENE McCOLLUM-FLANIGAN was born and reared in Conyers, Georgia, a small, but very rapidly growing town in the East Atlanta Metropolitan Area. She is the youngest child of five children of the late Arthur and Eula Bowden-McCollum.

She has a great feeling knowing that she has made positive influences and differences with adults and children in her chosen professions as a social worker and a public middle school teacher, Youth Sunday School teacher, wife, mother, grandmother, and a dependable friend and family member.

She has been creatively writing forever. upon retiring with a medical disability, she was spiritually guided to share personal and some embarrassing experiences that living with the chronic debilitating disease of multiple sclerosis causes one to bear.

"MULTIPLE SCLEROSIS, THE HORRENDOUS, NOTORIOUS, UNINVITED, INTRUDER", is her first published novel. However, she has two published poems copyrighted with the "National Poetry Society". She finds great enjoyment and peace with her family and friends. Her husband and her two adult sons and their families are exceptional loving people to her. She and her husband reside in their original hometown.

AUTHOR CONTACT INFORMATION

FOR MORE INFORMATION PLEASE CONTACT:

E. CARLENE McCOLLUM-FLANIGAN
PHONE: (770) 483-7347
WEBSITE: MAJRL5@BELLSOUTH.NET